SANITATION
without
WATER

by Uno Winblad and Wen Kilama
illustrations by Kjell Torstensson

i

An Arabic edition of this book is to be published by the WHO
Regional Office for Eastern Mediterranean, P.O. Box 1517,
ALEXANDRIA, Egypt.

Editions in French, Spanish and Portuguese are under pre-
paration. A simplified version of this book called "How to
Build a Compost Latrine" is to be published in Swahili,
Amharic and English in 1981. Requests for copies should be
addressed to SIDA, S-105 25 STOCKHOLM, Sweden, atten-
tion Health Division.

ACKNOWLEDGEMENT

The publication of this monograph was made possible by a grant from SIDA, the Swedish International Development Authority, Stockholm.

The research and development behind this book has been supported by a number of institutions over several years. The Scandinavian Institute of African Studies, Uppsala, provided a travel grant in 1970; DANIDA, the Danish International Development Agency, Copenhagen, awarded a research grant in 1971; IDRC, the International Development Research Centre, Ottawa, funded a comparative study of compost latrines in Tanzania 1974-1978, and a study tour to China in 1975; the Swedish Institute, Stockholm, contributed a travel grant in 1974; and the Tanzania National Scientific Research Council in cooperation with the Faculty of Medicine, University of Dar es Salaam, provided personnel, accommodation and laboratory facilities for field experiments and laboratory tests in 1975-1978, SIDA a travel grant in 1980, and the Ethiopian Science and Technology Commission a seminar in Ethiopia in 1980.

To all these institutions and to friends and colleagues who critically examined the preliminary edition the authors wish to express their sincere appreciation.

The views expressed in this book are those of the authors and do not necessarily represent those of the personnel within the institutions sponsoring the research, development and publication.

CONTENTS

In an economy of scarcity, the mass of the common
people, though poor, possess the bulk of the nation's
human and material resources for housing. Their
collective entrepreneurial and managerial skills
(and spare time) far surpass the financial and ad-
ministrative capacity of even the most highly plan-
ned and centralized institutional system - whether
dominated by the state or by private capitalist
corporations.

J.F.C. TURNER

INTRODUCTION

The flush toilet cannot solve the
problems of excreta disposal in
the poor countries. Nor has it
indeed solved those problems in
the rich part of the world. It is
expensive to install, uses large
amounts of clean water to flush
away excreta, and pollutes the
receiving stream, lake or aquifer.
For the large majority of the
world's population that still has
no access to piped water, a flush
toilet is not even an alternative
to consider.

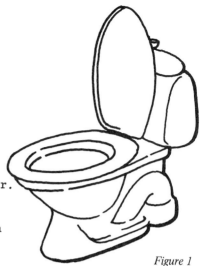

Figure 1

WHY IS EXCRETA DISPOSAL A PROBLEM?

Human faeces are potentially dangerous, malodorous, surrounded by taboos and expensive to dispose of.

A large number of diseases are spread directly through
man's contact with human excrement, indirectly via water,
food and soil, or via carriers and vectors like flies, cockroaches and mosquitoes. These dangers of poor sanitation
are augmented by increasing population densities. When
people move from isolated farms into villages and from
rural tracts into urban squatter areas, they may be better
off in a number of ways but certainly not with respect to
sanitation. Simple disposal systems like defecation in the
bush, in fields or in open pits may have no adverse effects
for small, scattered populations. But when used in densly
built up areas, such practices could be outright dangerous.

The potential nuisance from human excreta is too well known
to need elaboration: the noxious odours, the flies ...

1

Defecation practices are in some cultures surrounded by taboos. Those who empty buckets and clean latrines may be regarded as outcasts, men and women or parents and children may not be allowed to use the same latrine, an enemy who gets hold of your faeces can cause you great harm, bad spirits live in the pit ... Religion may lay down strict rules for the location and use of latrines or prescribe the application of water for anal cleansing.

Excreta disposal can be expensive, especially in urban areas. In most large cities in developing countries only the wealthy elite has a reasonably satisfactory disposal system. The wast majority has to make do with self-built, noxious and unsound latrines.

EXISTING SYSTEMS

There are basically two ways of dealing with human excreta: they can either be transported away for treatment or discharge, or disposed of on site. Whichever way is used, the excreta can either be mixed or not mixed with water. This gives us four possibilities:

	TRANSPORT	NO TRANSPORT
WATER	1. *flush toilet connected to sewer* *aqua privy connected to sewer*	3. *flush toilet connected to septic tank* *aqua privy* *cesspool* *biogas tank*
NO WATER	2. *bucket latrine* *long drop latrine*	4. *compost latrine* *pit latrine*

Figure 2

Transport is the most expensive item of group 1. Up to 80% of the total cost of flush toilet systems goes to the collection network. Such a network is not required for group 2, but the high costs of frequent bucket collection can make this system even more expensive in the long run. Bucket collection is common in China where the high costs are offset against the fertilizer value of human excreta (see Chapter 3 for a detailed description of this system). In group 3 we find systems often used in developing countries, at least for the more wealthy part of the population. In this group transport is required only for sludge removal. The most common systems here are septic tanks and aqua privies. They have a high failure rate as they are often installed where soil conditions are unsuitable for absorption of the effluent.

The systems belonging to the first three groups are well covered in conventional texts on public health engineering. This book therefore concentrates on group 4: dry systems for on site composting or disposal of excreta and organic residues. The well known and much abused traditional pit latrine belongs to this group as does the little known compost latrine.

The group 4 systems require neither transport nor water. Compost latrines can be used under the most difficult soil and ground water conditions. Pit latrines are not as adaptable, but where they can be built they are unsurpassed in simplicity and economy. A word of caution though: there are no miracle solutions to the problems of excreta disposal. Extravagant claims have been made, especially for compost latrines, in recent years. Inventors and manufacturers of various contraptions have maintained that their devices operate at "temperatures above 60°C" and thereby "completely destroy all pathogens", and that they are "odourfree" and "flyproof". It is not as simple as that. The methods and systems described on the following pages can work and some work very well indeed. But when not fully understood by the users or constructed in the wrong way or in the wrong place they may fail completely.

SANITATION WITHOUT WATER – IS IT FEASIBLE?

The failure or success of a latrine system depends on the interaction of three sets of factors: environmental, human and technical:

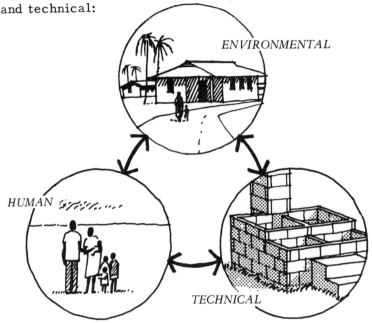

ENVIRONMENTAL

HUMAN

TECHNICAL

Figure 3

The most important environmental components are climate, soil, and ground water. They vary from one location to another and have a great influence on the type of latrine we may choose.

The foremost human element is motivation. If a man is motivated he will build a latrine and use it. Without motivation little can be achieved. The mere provision of a latrine is no guarantee that it will be used, or used properly. Motivation can be created by vigorous health education campaigns emphasizing the relation between insanitary practices and disease. This is not an easy matter to achieve in a community where the "bug-theory" of disease is not generally accepted. However, successful campaigns have been carried out in China and Vietnam with spectacular results for the health situation.

4

The technical components are variable. There is no particular design to suit all environmental and human conditions. The technology selected must be adapted to local environmental conditions, to the availability of financial resources, skills and materials, and whenever possible, to the customary "latrine behaviour" of the user.

ABOUT THIS BOOK

This book has been prepared to meet the increasing demand for practical information on how to design, build and operate compost latrines and improved pit latrines. The emphasis is on simple measures that can be implemented with limited resources.

We shall concentrate on sanitation systems for individual households. Public latrines for places like markets and railway stations and latrines for institutions like schools and hospitals are only mentioned briefly in this book. Some of the latrine systems described in the following chapters could possibly be adapted to public or institutional use. The problem there is not so much one of design and construction but rather of supervision, cleaning and maintenance.

Our aim has been to produce a simple, readable and well-illustrated manual primarily for health officers, sanitarians, medical auxiliaries and village technicians in Africa. It should also be of relevance to medical officers interested in disease prevention and to physical planners, architects, and civil and sanitary engineers concerned with appropriate technology.

The general background information and the examples should be useful also to readers outside Africa. With some adaptation to local conditions the technical solutions put forward in the concluding chapters may be applicable in other parts of the world.

The first part of the book contains two chapters with general background information on the relation between sanitation and disease and on the composting process. In Part II thirteen different dry sanitation systems from various parts of the world are described. They have been selected to demonstrate the range of technical solutions already in use. The choice is not as restricted as most textbooks on public health engine,- ering seem to imply! Part III is a manual. First comes a systematic presentation of latrine components. By using that information it should be possible to design latrines suitable for a great variety of situations. The following chapter in the manual is primarily intended for those who instruct self- builders and craftsmen. It gives a step-by-step account of how to select, locate and construct a latrine. Operating instructions are given in the last chapter and are very important - especially for those who have or are considering compost latrines. Finally there is an appendix on fly control in dry latrines - a most difficult problem for which there is as yet no satisfactory single solution.

FURTHER READING

FEACHEM, R. & CAIRNCROSS, S. (1978), *Small excreta disposal systems.* Ross Bulletin No 8. The Ross Institute of Tropical Hygiene, London.

RYBCZYNSKI, W., POLPRASERT, C. & McGARRY, M. (1978), *Low-cost technology options for sanitation.* IDRC, Ottawa.

STONER. C. H. ed. (1977), *Goodbye to the flush toilet.* Rodale Press Inc, Emmaus, Pa.

WINBLAD, U. (1972), *Evaluation of waste disposal systems for urban low income communities in Africa.* Scan Plan Report No 3/1972, Copenhagen.

Chapter 1

SANITATION AND DISEASE

Numerous infections and infestations of man are spread
through inadequate sanitation. Viruses, bacteria, and parasites may spread through direct contact, indirectly via food,
water and soil, or via carriers and vectors.

In this chapter we shall look at the common routes of transmission, mention the most important diseases associated
with insanitary conditions and outline preventive measures.
Symptoms and treatments are not discussed here as information of that kind is readily available in medical textbooks.

INFECTION FROM INGESTION OF FOOD OR DRINK CONTAMINATED WITH FAECES

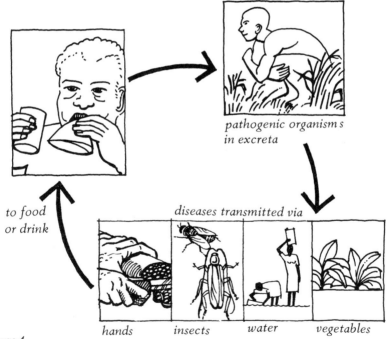

pathogenic organisms in excreta

to food or drink

diseases transmitted via

hands insects water vegetables

Figure 4

Viral diseases like poliomyelitis and infectious hepatitis, bacterial diseases like cholera, salmonella, shigella and bacillary dysentery, protozoal diseases like amoebic dysentery and giardiasis, and worm infections like ascariasis and trichuriasis are transmitted through faecally contaminated food or drink.

The modern control of poliomyelitis is based on vaccination of infants and children. For all the other diseases mentioned above, the most important measure is the sanitary disposal of human faeces and protection of food and water supplies. The control of filth flies is essential (a variety of methods are discussed in the Appendix to this book) and food should be protected from flies and cockroaches. Health education stressing personal hygiene and sanitary handling of food and drinking water must be given a high priority.

INFECTION FROM INGESTION OF BEEF OR PORK INFECTED WITH TAPEWORM

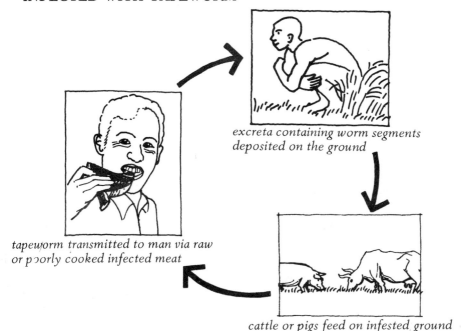

excreta containing worm segments deposited on the ground

tapeworm transmitted to man via raw or poorly cooked infected meat

cattle or pigs feed on infested ground

Figure 5

8

The most important tapeworms of man are transmitted to him via cattle and pigs. An infected man passes worm segments in his faeces. When the segments disintegrate they release eggs. Cattle or pigs feeding on infested grounds ingest the eggs, which undergo development in their muscles. Man aquires the infection by eating raw or undercooked infected meat. Under suitable environmental conditions eggs may remain viable in pastures for eight or more weeks.

The prevention of tapeworm infections demands proper disposal of human faeces so that neither cattle nor pigs have access to them. It is therefore important in health education to emphasize the dangers of contaminating soil or water with human excreta. Health education must also stress that all meat has to be thoroughly cooked. The treatment of infected individuals may reduce the source of animal infection.

INFECTION FROM CONTACT WITH WATER

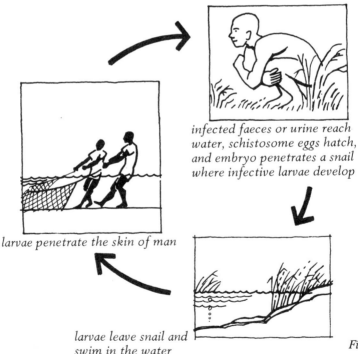

infected faeces or urine reach water, schistosome eggs hatch, and embryo penetrates a snail where infective larvae develop

larvae penetrate the skin of man

larvae leave snail and swim in the water

Figure 6

9

The major disease transmitted via infected water is schistosomiasis (bilharziasis). It is caused by blood flukes mainly belonging to one of the species *Schistosoma haematobium, S. mansoni*
and *S. japonicum*. The first one causes urinary schistosomiasis
and the other two intestinal schistosomiasis.

S. mansoni is essentially an African species although the slave
trade is claimed to have extended its range to the Arabian
peninsula and to tropical America including the West Indies.
S. haematobium is restricted to Africa and *S. japonicum* to the
Orient.

Man pollutes water with infected urine or stool containing
schistosome eggs. The eggs hatch in water and the resulting
larvae penetrate certain freshwater snails where they eventually develop into infective larvae. The process inside the
snail takes three or four weeks. The snail sheds the larvae
(less than 1 mm long) and man aquires the infection while
bathing, swimming, washing, fishing, cultivating or collecting aquatic plants in infested waters. Outside the snail the
larvae have at most two days to find a human being. The infection is from penetration of the skin by the infective larvae.

The control of schistosomiasis is difficult and the disease is
increasing in many parts of the developing world. The drugs
currently available are expensive, not fully effective, and
treatment may be accompanied by bad side effects. Moreover,
the few eggs not cleared by tretment are capable of giving
rise to a multitude of infective larvae which may continue the
transmission.

Snail vectors may be killed with molluscicides but such treatment is expensive and beyond the financial capabilities of most
affected communities. Besides, molluscicides are toxic to
man and to other non-target animals and plants.

The provision of an adequate and safe water supply would
reduce exposure to infected waters but has little effect where
people fish, work in irrigated fields or collect water plants.

The safe disposal of human excreta is an essential measure
in combating schistosomiasis. The success of this approach
depends on people accepting the use of latrines. Since schisto-

somiasis control is so difficult and intricate, its proper implementation must rely on the integration of various measures with great emphasis on environmental sanitation.

INFECTION FROM CONTACT WITH SOIL

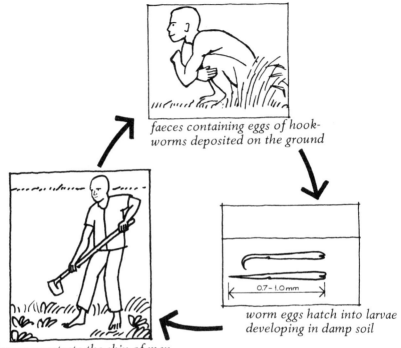

faeces containing eggs of hook-worms deposited on the ground

worm eggs hatch into larvae developing in damp soil

larvae penetrate the skin of man

Figure 7

Certain parasitic worms such as hookworms and *Strongyloides stercoralis* penetrate the skin from damp soil contaminated with human faeces. The hookworm eggs are discharged with faeces from infected persons. They hatch into larvae which feed on organic debris and bacteria. Under optimal environmental conditions they develop into infective larvae in about one week and remain viable for up to five weeks. After penetrating the skin, the larvae migrate through man's body and eventually mature in his intestines after 4-7 weeks.

Many drugs are available for the treatment of hookworm infection but treated patients are often reinfected immediately

11

they return to their hookworm infested communities. The control of hookworms must again emphasize sanitary disposal of faeces. The integration of environmental sanitation with mass treatment reinforced by health education campaigns is a necessary combination for good results.

The development of *S. stercoralis* generally parallels that of hookworms. However, treatment of *S. stercoralis* is not easy and the drugs currently available may give rise to unpleasant effects. The best control method is the safe disposal of human faeces. The parasite may survive outside man, for instance in a latrine, for a considerable length of time. It is therefore essential to avoid unnecessary handling of faeces, even those that have been composted.

INFECTION VIA INSECT VECTORS

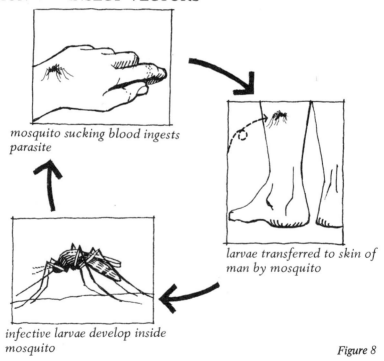

mosquito sucking blood ingests parasite

larvae transferred to skin of man by mosquito

infective larvae develop inside mosquito

Figure 8

Among the diseases indirectly related to excreta disposal, Bancroftian filariasis is an important one. The end result of this disease is elephantiasis and a host of abnormalities among which are extreme swelling of genital organs. Bancroftian filariasis is caused by a parasite, called *Wuchereria bancrofti*. The transmission of this infection requires a suitable species of mosquito. The principal vector throughout the urbanizing tropical and subtropical world is *Culex quinquefasciatus* (previously known as *Culex pipiens fatigans*). The parasites are ingested by the blood-sucking mosquito where they develop into infective filariform larvae. The infective larvae are transferred to man while the mosquito is biting.

The transmission of filariasis is only indirectly related to excreta disposal. Where the disposal of wastes, including excreta, is faulty the breeding of *C. quinquefasciatus* increases. This mosquito breeds in foul waters; its juvenile aquatic stages are therefore abundant in ditches, drains, gulley-traps, cesspits, faulty septic tanks, aqua privies, pit latrines, and any other accumulation of water with a high content of organic matter. The rapid growth of unplanned, poorly serviced urban and periurban areas in Africa, Asia and Latin America has led to tremendous increases in *C. quinquefasciatus* mosquito populations. As a consequence there is increased transmission and prevalence of Bancroftian filariasis.

This *Culex* mosquito can be controlled with insecticides, but it is a method with many limitations. The cost is extremely high, mosquitoes often develop insecticide resistance, insecticides are toxic to man and to other animals. The risk for water pollution is high as the insecticides currently available have to be applied repeatedly to mosquito breeding water. Insecticidal control of adult *C. quinquifasciatus* is of very limited value.

The individual may protect himself with mosquito repellents, bed nets, screened houses, and protective clothing. At the community level the most important preventive measure is to avoid creating breeding habitats. Latrines should be dry - they must not reach down into the ground water. Cesspools, aqua privies and septic tanks must be perfectly sealed.

Another serious limitation in the current methods of filariasis control is the lack of satisfactory drugs for either individual or mass protection against this disease.

CONCLUSIONS

There are no shortcuts to improved public health in developing countries. Vaccination, chemotherapy and insecticides are in most cases of limited value. Lasting results can only be achieved with the general introduction of satisfactory systems for water supply, waste-water disposal and sanitation together with intensive health education campaigns.

Chapter 2

COMPOSTING

BASIC PRINCIPLES

Composting is a biological process in which various types of organisms under controlled conditions break down organic substances to a humus end product (mature compost). It is the "controlled conditions" which distinguish a composting operation from a garbage heap or manure pile.

Decomposition of organic matter by biological action has been taking place in nature since life first appeared on earth. The organisms required for this decomposition are available in organic materials and do not have to be added.

The art of composting for turning human and animal excrement and plant residues into fertilizer was known to many ancient civilizations, notably that of China. In his "Book of Agriculture" written in the 12th century Ibn-al Awam of Seville gives details of how to prepare a compost with human excreta as the major ingredient. The method he used 800 years ago was similar to the one still used in China and described in the following chapter.

The simplest method of composting, in heaps or windrows (elongated heaps) in the open air, is still widely used by gardeners.

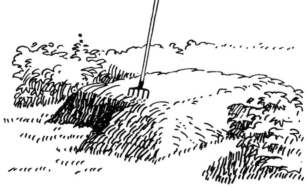

Figure 9

15

The compost is built up gradually: layer upon layer of grass clippings, weeds, all kinds of garden debris and organic household residues form the heap. For quicker decomposition it may be turned after a week or two and again after a month, or the heap can be built with air channels as often done in China. Neither turning nor air channels are absolutely necessary. Good results can be achieved without it (Bruce 1967). Depending on the number of turnings, the season, and the raw material in the heap the compost may take from four weeks to several months to mature.

Composting is a biological process and is thus influenced by a number of environmental factors such as aeration, temperature, moisture, pH value, and the ratio of carbon to nitrogen (C/N ratio).

Aeration

Some of the microbes need oxygen to carry on the decomposition. Such organisms are said to be aerobic. Others do not require oxygen - they are called anaerobic. Many organisms can be either anaerobic or aerobic depending on the environment. Oxygen is taken from the air surrounding or trapped inside the compost heap.

Composting processes are often classified as either aerobic or anaerobic but both types are actually going on at the same time in a compost heap. Near the surface the process may be aerobic while in the interior it is anaerobic.

Aerobic conditions are necessary for rapid, odourfree decomposition and for destruction of pathogenic organisms by heat. Absence of air will lead to different types of micro-organisms developing. Under such conditions decomposition is slower, foul smelling gases (hydrogen sulphide and ammonia) are released and the heat given off is only a fraction of that from aerobic composting.

The most common way of aerating a compost heap is by turning. A simple device for turning the heap in a compost latrine is described in Chapter 4. Another method of aeration is to provide air channels right through the heap as shown in the example from China and Sweden in the next chapter. Earth-

16

worms and insects also play an important role in aerating the compost heap. Special aeration devices are therefore usually not necessary especially since only small amounts of oxygen are required to maintain aerobic conditions.

Temperature

Considerable amounts of heat are released by aerobic decomposition. If the heap is large enough much of it is retained due to the insulating properties of the compost material. With the mass large enough and other conditions favourable, the temperature inside the heap can reach 70°C. But in a compost latrine temperatures above 50°C are rarely reached. When this happens the high temperature is restricted to a small part of the pile.

Decomposition within the temperature range from 10°C up to around 45°C is carried out by so called mesophilic microorganisms. At temperatures above 45°C the process is taken over by thermophilic micro-organisms.

Conditions favouring decomposition at temperatures above 45°C are: large bulk (at least 0.5-1.0 cu m), low moisture content (50-60%), large input of green grass, weeds and kitchen residues (four or five times the amount of faeces), chopped or crushed raw material, and occasional turning.

Moisture

All organisms require water for life but too high moisture content in the compost heap may give rise to anaerobic conditions. This is because the material becomes soggy, compact and unable to contain sufficient air in the spaces between the particles. A very low content of water on the other hand retards the activity of the microbes. In a compost latrine the best results in terms of pathogen destruction are achieved with a moisture content of 50-60%.

An extremely wet latrine could be the result of a combination of some of the following factors: humid climate, water used for anal cleansing, urine as well as faeces deposited, too many users, no addition of organic refuse, unventilated receptacle, entry of rain-, surface- or ground water.

The other extreme could result from a dry climate, use of paper or dry leaves for anal cleansing, collection of urine separately and seepage of liquid into the subsoil.

Acidity or pH value

The acidity/alkalinity of the compost is expressed by the hydrogen ion concentration on the so called pH scale. The scale runs from 0 to 14. Figure 7 stands for neutrality, higher values indicate alkalinity and the lower ones acidity. The best pH range for most bacteria is from 6 to 7.5 and for fungi from 5.5 to 8.

Fresh human excreta are slightly acid (pH value less than 7) but after a few days in a compost heap the pH usually begins to rise. Latrine contents are therefore normally alkaline. Highly alkaline conditions will lead to excessive loss of nitrogen in the form of ammonia. The amount lost can be reduced by adding a little soil, about 1% of the weight of the heap, well mixed with the other ingredients. If the process turns anaerobic, large amounts of organic acid are produced, thus lowering the pH. The addition of wood ashes or lime will increase the pH. Normally there is no necessity to influence the pH of a compost latrine.

Ratio of carbon to nitrogen

Microbes feed on organic matter containing, among other things, carbon and nitrogen. They use carbon for energy and nitrogen for body building. The carbon/nitrogen balance in a compost or soil is called the C/N ratio. The microbes require much more carbon than nitrogen: the optimum C/N ratio for composting is thus within the range 15/1 and 30/1 in the initial mixture.

Excreta and especially urine are rich in nitrogen. The C/N ratio of human faeces is around 8/1 and of urine 0.8/1. Green grass clippings and vegetable trimmings have a C/N ratio of about 15/1 while straw and sawdust are very low in nitrogen, with a ratio for straw of about 150/1 and for sawdust up to 500/1.

18

The more the C/N ratio differs from the optimum range of from 15/1 to 30/1, the slower the decomposition proceeds. To achieve quick decomposition in a latrine it is therefore necessary to add high carbon materials like grass, garden litter, sawdust, and organic household and kitchen residue. Excluding urine from the latrine (as the Vietnamese do, see Chapter 3) would have a similar effect.

LIFE IN THE COMPOST HEAP

An immense variety of organisms are living in and contributing to the break down of the compost heap. They range in size from viruses, bacteria, fungi and algae to earthworms, arthropods and rodents. It is this rich fauna and flora that is responsible for the rapid decomposition taking place in a well functioning compost latrine.

The bigger organisms play a limited role in the decomposition process in a large composting plant and are not able to survive the high temperatures (60°-70°C) of a garden compost that is turned frequently. The conditions in a compost latrine are more favourable to higher animals as the temperature normally does not exceed 40°-45°C.

Fly maggots, earthworms, snails, slugs, ants, mites, spiders, sowbugs, beetles, and cockroaches play a major role in mixing, aerating and tearing apart the contents of the latrine. As long as they remain inside the receptacle their activities are beneficial and should be encouraged. It might even be a good idea to place earthworms like the redworm *(Eisenia foetida)* and the nightcrawler *(Lumbricus terrestris)* in the latrine. If the environment is favourable for them they will multiply, burrowing holes through the compost heap, eating odorous organic matter and thereby converting it into rich organic soil.

Most of the invertebrate inhabitants of the latrine are harmless to man, but there are some we do not like to see outside: the filth fly, the *Culex* mosquito and the cockroach are obvious examples. The possibility of controlling these insects is

19

discussed elsewhere in this book.

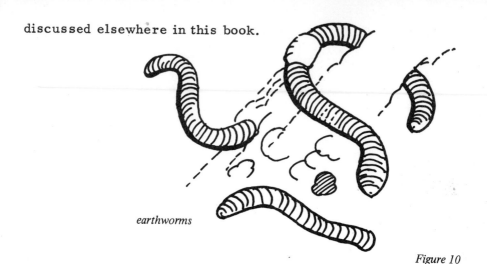

earthworms

Figure 10

Although many of the organisms are present on the raw
materials, the addition of some partly decomposed material
from an existing compost heap to a new heap will accelerate
the process by introducing acclimatized micro-organisms.

DESTRUCTION OF PATHOGENIC ORGANISMS

Once the excreta have been deposited in a compost latrine they
remain there for a long time: from two months up to several
years depending on the system used. Sooner or later the
latrine has to be emptied or closed down. If it is to be
emptied: How safe are the contents in terms of the potential
spread of disease?

High temperature composting can effectively destroy pathogenic organisms but, as has been shown previously, high
temperatures are not likely in a compost latrine. Temperatures above 50°C, if reached, do not last long, and are likely
to be restricted to only part of the pile.

The destruction of pathogenic organisms by high temperature
alone can therefore not be relied upon in a latrine. Fortunately

other factors in the compost environment contribute to the destruction of pathogens: time, unfavourable pH value, competition for nutrient, antibiotic action, toxic by-products of decomposing organisms, and anaerobic conditions.

After six months in a closed receptacle the contents of a well functioning compost latrine can be considered safe enough to be taken out, placed in a shallow trench and covered with soil. Most parasitic organisms have been destroyed and the amount of faecal coliform organisms reduced to the level normally found in the soil. Parasites like *Strongyloides stercoralis* and *Ascaris lumbricoides* des can however survive the composting process and handling of compost should therefore be reduced to a minimum.

COMPOST AS A FERTILIZER AND SOIL CONDITIONER

Compost is vital to the health of growing plants. Its main value is as a soil conditioner, providing whatever may be lacking in the physical and chemical makeup of the soil. This is particularly important for tropical soils which are often low in organic content. Addition of compost will make the soil easier to cultivate and improves its water holding capacity, thus helping to prevent cracking and erosion by wind and water.

Compost from the "multrum" described in Chapter 3 has an organic content of 58% (on a dry weight basis). The percentage of major plant nutrients - nitrogen, phosphorus, and potassium - can be as high as 2.4%, 3.6%, and 3.9% respectively. This means that about 3 kg dry weight (about 10 kg "wet" weight) is roughly equivalent to 1 kg of "10-10-10" fertilizer. In addition the compost contains significant amounts of the minor plant nutrients calcium, magnesium and sulphur, as well as a variety of trace elements and microbes (Fogel 1977). The major plant nutrients as well as the trace elements are fixed in organic compounds. Therefore in spite of the relatively low percentage of nutrient contents in compost, their utilization by plants can be close to 100%. Chemical fertilizers, on the other hand, are water soluble and will to a large extent be washed into ground water, streams and lakes. A high percentage of the nutrients in chemical fertilizers are therefore not utilized by the plants.

The amount of major plant nutrients ("N-P-K") available to developing countries through organic residues and nightsoil was in 1971 seven or eight times larger than their actual consumption of manufactured fertilizers (FAO/SIDA 1975). Few countries are systematically making use of this treasure - the notable exceptions being China and Vietnam.

"Wastes" is obviously a misleading term for excreta, kitchen refuse, sweepings, and crop and garden leavings. The rest of the world could learn from the Chinese to regard these residual products as valuable resources. The term "waste" should be replaced by "residue".

REFERENCES CITED

BRUCE, M. E. (1967), *Common sense compost making.* Faber & Faber, London.

FOA/SIDA (1975), *Organic materials as fertilizer.* Soils Bulletin No 27, Rome.

FOGEL, M. (1977), Chemical analysis of Clivus Multrum compost. Clivus Multrum USA Inc, Cambridge, Mass. (mimeo).

FURTHER READING

COOPER, R. C. & GOLUEKE, C. G. (1977), Public health aspects of on-site waste treatment. Compost Science 18(3):8-11.

DALZELL, H. W., GRAY, K. R. & BIDDLESTONE, A. J. (1979), *Composting in tropical agriculture.* International Institute of Biological Husbandry, Ipswich, Suffolk, UK.

GOLUEKE, C. G. (1975), *Composting – a study of the process and its principles.* Rodale Press Inc. Emmaus, Pa, USA.

GOTAAS, H. B. (1956), *Composting – sanitary disposal and reclamation of organic wastes.* WHO Monograph Series No 31, Geneva.

HILLS, L. D. (1975), *Fertility without fertilizers.* Henry Doubleday Research Association, Bocking, UK.

VOORHOEVE, J. J. C. (1974), *Organic fertilizers – problems and potential for developing countries.* World Bank Fertilizer Study, Background Paper No 4, Washington D.C.

Chapter 3

EXAMPLES OF SANITATION WITHOUT WATER

INTRODUCTION

In this chapter we discuss and comment on thirteen systems of excreta disposal from various parts of the world. The selection has been made in order to represent a wide variety of cultural, environmental and economic conditions.

Culturally the most important distinction in this context is between those who regard human excreta as a valuable resource and those who view it as an unpleasant and dangerous waste product. The former concept leads to composting (examples from China, Vietnam, India, Algeria, and Sweden) while the latter results in a final disposal system (Tanzania, Zimbabwe, S. Africa, Egypt, and USA).

We have included systems suitable for areas where the ground water table is low and systems that can be used under any ground water conditions. The selection includes examples from urban areas with very high housing density as well as from low density rural areas, rich countries as well as poor countries.

The example from China is an illustration of proper composting. Its disadvantage is that fresh excreta have to be transported. This is also the case with the systems from Yemen and Algeria. Although drying and decomposition take place in the receptacle there is still some handling of fresh excreta. The examples from Vietnam, India, and Sweden describe real compost latrines: the decomposition takes place in the receptacle. No handling is required until the excreta have been transformed into non-offensive, less harmfull humus.

The chapter also contains five examples of pit latrines. Tanzania illustrates the "final disposal" approach: excreta are deposited in a deep pit from where they are not usually removed. The examples from USA, Egypt, Zimbabwe, and S. Africa are variations on the same theme.

23

None of the prefabricated, compact type of toilets which are now sold in the Scandinavian countries and in N. America has been included in this chapter. They are too expensive and too complex to be considered for large scale use in developing countries.

CHINA: "Four into One" composting

Composting of human and animal excreta has been practised in China for thousands of years. In 1952 an estimated 70% of all human excreta produced in China were collected and used as fertilizer. In 1956 this figure had been pushed up to an unbelievable 90%, altogether some 300 million tons (Dorozynski 1975). At the time that represented about one third of all fertilizers applied in the country.

In rural areas the latrine was often combined with a pig-pen in such a way that the pigs could feed on human excreta.

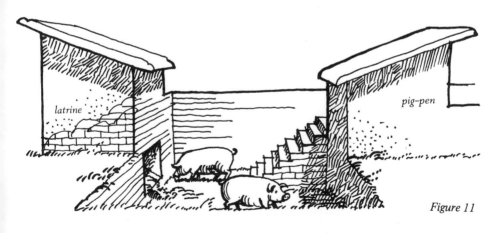

latrine

pig-pen

Figure 11

24

This practice is now discouraged both because it is considered unhygienic and because some of the fertilizer value of the human excreta is lost. Existing combined latrine/pig-pen units are rebuilt and the latrine separated from the pen and turned into a "shallow pit". The pit is emptied daily and its contents brought to a compost station where they are mixed with animal manure, refuse and soil.

The "shallow pit" is normally designed for separation of faeces and urine. The urine is collected in a jar placed either directly in front of the latrine as in this picture or drained away via a channel to a urine pit or a jar at some distance away from the latrine.

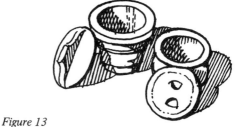

Figure 12

The "shallow pit" is no more than 0.10 - 0.15 m deep. With a "deep pit" the Chinese generally mean one that is 0.40 - 0.50 m. "Shallow pits" are preferred because they are easier to empty and keep clean.

Bucket latrines are still in common use in China. The buckets are often made from wood and beautifully laquered.

Figure 13

The contents of buckets and pits are carried or wheeled to the compost station in willow baskets, pails or other containers, often transported on special tricycles.

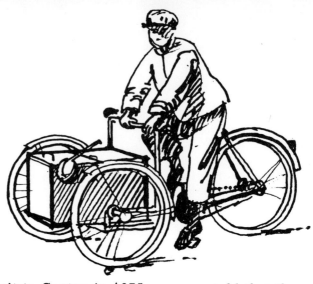

Figure 14

During a study visit to Canton in 1975 we were told that the
collection of excreta in that city used to be controlled by un-
scrupoluos racketeers who sold the excreta to peasants.
These practices were stopped after the liberation and a
special organization was set up to collect, treat and distri-
bute all household residues. After the collectivization movement in 1956 peasants started coming into Canton to do their
own collection. As many as 15,000 commune members would
enter the city every night, empty the latrines and buckets and
carry the treasure back to the villages. Leaking containers
and careless handling caused spilling and unsanitary conditions.
The collection has now been reorganized and is carried out by
salaried sanitary workers. In 1975 the communes around
Canton paid from Yuan 3.40 to 5.58 per ton for nightsoil -
exact price depending on water content. (Normal wages at the
time were Yuan 60-70 per month.)

The purpose of the treatment at the station is to destroy pathogens without loss of fertilizer value. Various methods are
used, ranging from anaerobic fermentation in tanks to aerobic
composting in heaps or pits.

A common method is "Four into One" high temperature composting (McGarry & Stainforth 1978). Four types of raw
material are used: human excreta, animal manure, soil, and
street sweepings.

Roughly equal proportions of the four types of raw material are mixed and piled 0.15 m high. Water is added if necessary.

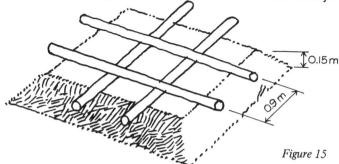

0.15 m

0.9 m

Four pieces of timber of 70 - 100 mm diameter (or a bundle of millet stalks) are placed on top of the pile as shown here. The distance between timbers is about 0.9 m.

At the crossing points four vertical pieces of the same dimensions are erected.

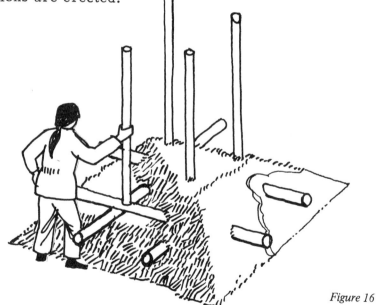

Figure 16

Raw material is piled up to a height of 0.9 m and covered with a 50 mm soil/manure mix (two thirds soil, one third manure). The earth covering serves several purposes: it

27

prevents rainwater from soaking the pile, reduces evaporation, lessens loss of nitrogen, checks fly breeding and odours,
and increases the surface temperature.

When the covering mix has dried, the timber pieces are
pulled out.

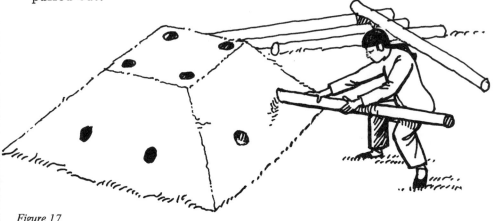

Figure 17

Air movement through the holes keeps the decomposition
process aerobic. In spring and autumn the holes are blocked
at night to prevent cooling. In summer when compost temperatures reach 50°C the holes are blocked to check evaporation rate and nitrogen loss. In winter the piles are often
built without holes.

In wintertime the humidity of the compost is kept at around
30%, in late spring and early summer it should be around
40%, and in summer it is raised to about 50%. A skilled
compost operator is able to estimate the humidity from poking
the pile with a stick.

Compost temperatures usually increase to 50°C-60°C. After
20 days in summer and up to 60 days in winter the crude
compost has matured and is ready for application on the fields.

The urine that was collected separately can be added to the
compost but more commonly it is diluted with water (1 part
urine to 5 parts water) and used directly on vegetable plots.

*The Chinese method of composting excreta with refuse is ecologically sound:
it causes no pollution of streams and lakes, and the discharges of faecal matter into ground water and soil should be well within the self-regenerative ca-
pability of the environment. Humus and nutrients removed by intensive cul-
tivation are returned to the soil.*

*From a health point of view it is doubtful though. Buckets and "shallow
pits" are emptied and cleaned daily and their contents are transported. This
means a lot of handling of fresh excreta, risk of spilling, and ample opportu-
nities for flies to gain access to faeces. The Chinese have, however, a long experience of handling excreta and the general standard of hygiene is such that
they are nowadays able to cope with the health hazards.*

*The running costs of this system ought to be high considering the large input
of labour for collection, transport and composting. But in China these costs
are offset by the even higher value put on the excreta.*

VIETNAM: the double-vault latrine

In parts of Vietnam, like in China, it used to be common
practice to fertilize rice fields with fresh excreta. In other
parts of the country "People were in the habit of relieving
themselves in the fields or at the sides of the less frequented
roads, leaving their excreta for sustenance for the famished
dogs" (McMichael 1976).

In 1956 the health authorities of the Democratic Republic of
Vietnam started campaigns for the construction of latrines.
After many experiments "the double septic tank for on-the-
spot composting of excreta" was developed by peasants in the
Quang Ngai Province. (To avoid confusion we shall not use
the term "septic tank" for this dry, double-vault latrine.)

In its first five year plan (1961-1965) the Ministry of Health
concentrated on what it called "the three major installations
for rural hygiene", namely the double-vault latrine, the lined
well, and the bathroom.

29

The Vietnamese latrine consists of two receptacles, each
with a volume of about 300 litres.

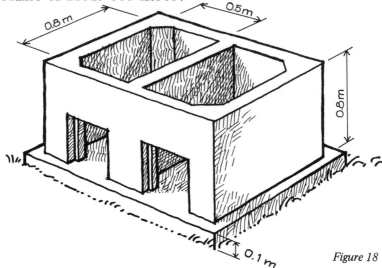

Figure 18

It is built entirely above ground with the two receptacles
placed on a solid floor of concrete, bricks or clay. The floor
must be at least 0.1 m above ground, so as not to be flooded
by heavy rains. The latrine should be located at least 10 m
away from dwelling houses and water tanks.

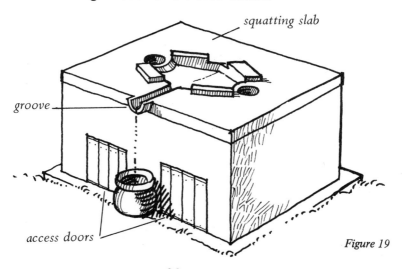

squatting slab

groove

access doors

Figure 19

30

The receptacles are covered with a squatting slab which has two holes, footrests and a channel for urine. Both holes are provided with tight fitting lids (not shown on the figures). In front there are steps leading up to the squatting slab, at the back there are two openings, 0.3 x 0.3 m, for the removal of the mature compost. These openings are kept sealed until one of the receptacles is to be emptied.

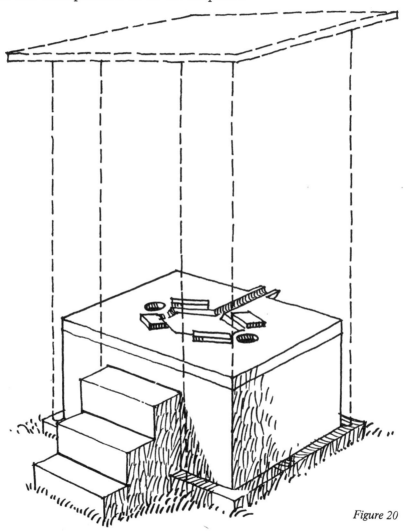

Figure 20

Faeces are deposited in one of the receptacles. Before it is used for the first time, the bottom is covered with a layer of powdered earth. The purpose of this earth is to absorb moisture from the faeces, to prevent them from sticking to the floor, and also to provide some of the micro-organisms for the decomposition process. After each use, two bowls of ashes are sprinkled over the faeces. The ashes absorb moisture, neutralize bad odours, and make the faeces less attractive to flies. (A ventpipe is said to serve no useful purpose as the ashes efficiently deodorize the latrine.)

Urine is drained away via the groove in the slab and collected in a jar behind the latrine. Input into the receptacle is thus only faeces, ashes and toilet paper. The contents are therefore fairly dry and compact and the decomposition process, according to Vietnamese sources (DRV, Ministry of Health 1968), basically anaerobic.

The receipient for urine can be an empty jar, a jar partly filled with water or a jar filled with ashes.

The first receptacle can be used for about two months by a household of 5-10 persons. When it is two thirds full, its contents are levelled with a stick and the receptacle is filled to the brim with dried, powdered earth. The first vault is then sealed (all openings tightly closed with lime mortar or clay) and the other one is used instead. When after another two months the second vault is nearly full, the first one is opened and emptied.

The temperature inside the vault is normally 2° to $6^{\circ}C$ higher than outside. In summer while the outside temperature is $28^{\circ}C$ to $32^{\circ}C$ the temperature inside a closed vault may come close to $50^{\circ}C$.

Around the latrine the Vietnamese grow insect repellant plants like citronella and *Acilepis squarosa*.

The Vietnamese health authorities claim that after 45 days in a sealed receptacle "all bacteria and pathogenic viruses, all eggs and embryos of intestinal parasites are killed, and toxic organic matters mineralized" (McMichael 1976).

32

The decomposed faeces, now odourless, provide an excellent fertilizer. Experiments carried out in agricultural cooperatives in Vietnam show that human excreta composted in double-vault latrines increases the yield of crops by 10% to 25% in comparison with fresh excreta (DRV, Ministry of Health 1968).

This system is now widely used in rural areas all over the country. In her book "Health in the Third World" Dr Joan McMichael (1976) states that of all the public health measures put into operation by the Vietnamese, the double-vault latrine has perhaps been the single most important factor in the prevention of disease and the promotion of health:

> "It strikes at the root cause of many of the most intractable diseases of the developing countries — the gastro-intestinal infections, cholera, dysentery and the typhoids — and checks the menace of fly borne infections. Last but perhaps no less important, it solves, in part at least, the problems of fertilizing the soil, since the yearly amount of sterilized organic manure that can thus be obtained is estimated at 600 000 tons."

These achievements have been reached after long and persistent health education campaigns. The task was not easy: some people found the latrine too expensive and complicated; in the North the peasants were convinced that manuring with fresh faeces was better than with composted ones; in certain villages people did not use the latrines in the correct way, which caused odours and heavy fly breeding; in some cases both vaults were used, one by men and the other by women (DRV, Ministry of Health 1968).

The Vietnamese system does not put any strain on the ecological balance of the environment as there are no discharges of excreta into water bodies, ground water or soil. When the excreta are finally returned to the soil they have already been transformed into humus through the decomposition taking place in the receptacle.

Most compost latrine systems require a considerable input of non-faecal organic refuse to achieve a favourable C/N ratio (see Chapter 2). The Vietnamese add only ashes, toilet paper and soil. The C/N ratio of the latrine contents is increased by the exclusion of urine from the receptacle.

From a health point of view the system should be acceptable provided the urine is taken care of in such a way that it does not reach fresh water. There is no handling of faeces, and fly breeding can be kept down as long as each user sprinkles ashes over his deposits. Two months' retention period seems to be on the short side though. The longer the faeces are stored, the less is the risk that pathogenic organisms survive.

The receptacles are built entirely above ground which means that they are dry — hence no breeding of Culex mosquitoes.

The construction is simple and the latrine can be built entirely from locally available materials. (The Vietnamese sources do not mention the corrosive effect of urine on concrete. This might be a problem.)

INDIA: the "gopuri" and the "sopa sandas" compost latrines

The most common system of excreta disposal in India is still indiscriminate defecation. With very few exceptions human faeces have never been used directly in agriculture.

Various types of latrines have been developed, amongst them a double-vault type, the "gopuri" latrine, similar to the Vietnamese model just described. There are some important differences though: the "gopuri" latrine has a permeable bottom, it has a ventpipe, and the input consists of household residue and urine as well as faeces.

Materials such as dry earth, ash, paddyhusks or hay are used for covering the excreta in the receptacle.

Another difference with the Vietnamese type is that the "gopuri" has two separate slabs, one for each vault. One is a proper squatting slab with a hole, the other one is a cover consisting of a piece of sheet metal. The hole in the squatting slab is covered with a lid when the latrine is not in use.

34

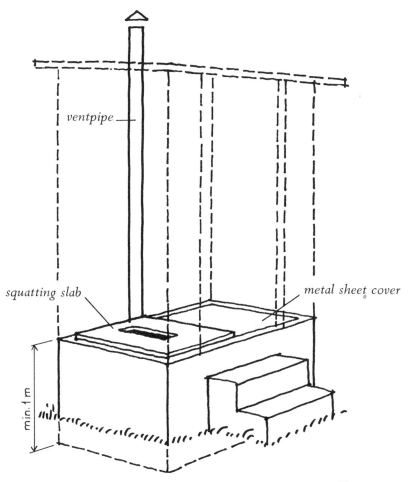

ventpipe

squatting slab

metal sheet cover

min. 1 m

Figure 21

When the first receptacle is filled to within two-thirds of its height, the slabs are shifted and the input deposited in the second vault (India, CPHERI 1964).

The "sopa sandas" type is an interesting variation of the "gopuri" latrine. The receptacle is not located under the squatting slab but is placed on the side. The hole and the receptacle are connected via a chute like in the S. African type described at the end of this chapter.

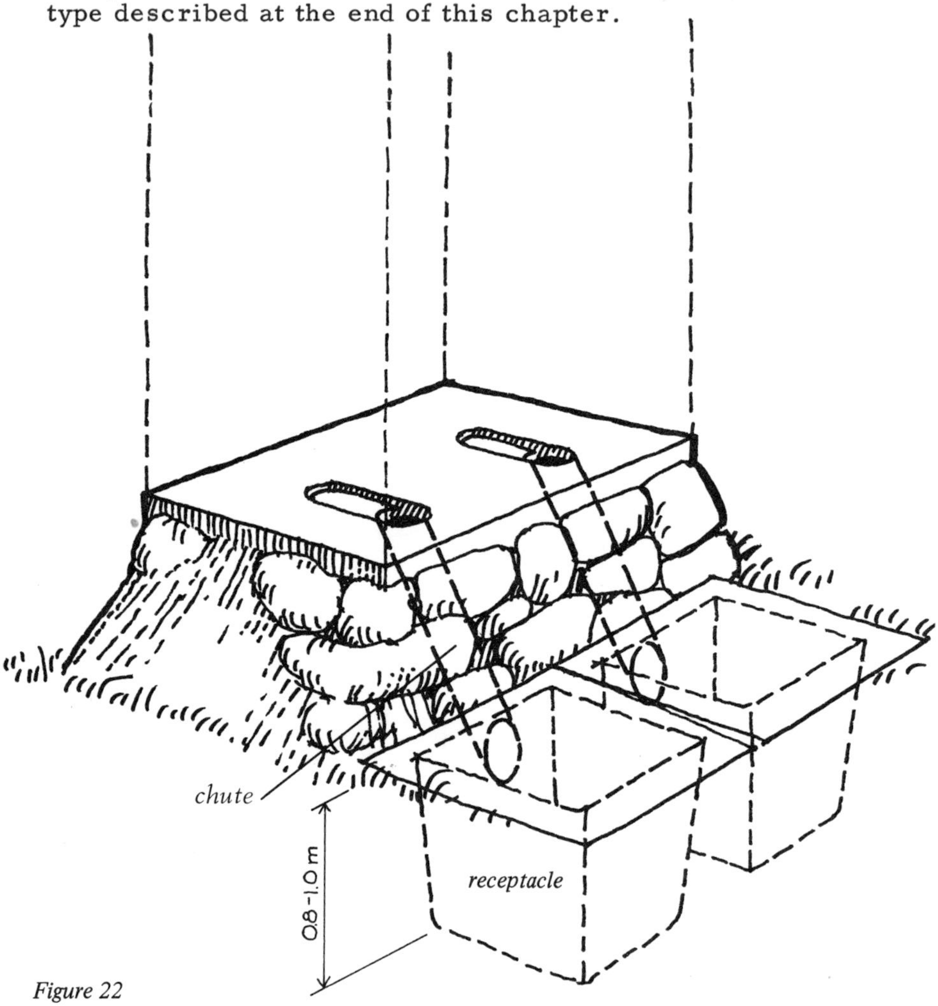

Figure 22

chute

0,8-1,0 m

receptacle

At the receptacle end the chute is covered with a flap-trap, a hinged lid, preventing insects and rodents from entering the vault, or if they are inside, from leaving it.

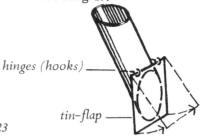

hinges (hooks)

tin-flap

Figure 23

The receptacle is a shallow, excavated pit divided into two chambers, each covered with a metal sheet. The metal sheet is removed when the receptacle is to be emptied (India, CPHERI 1964).

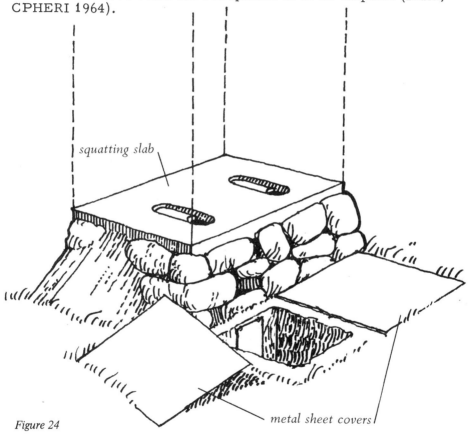

squatting slab

metal sheet covers

Figure 24

37

Both the "gopuri" and the "sopa sandas" latrines are ecologically sound. The amount of liquid seeping out from the receptacle and into the subsoil is small (if the latrine is used properly) and not likely to overtax the soil's ability for self regeneration.

There is no handling of faeces or urine, but fly breeding could be a problem with the "gopuri" type.

The "sopa sandas" is better in this respect. The flap-trap prevents flies from escaping from the receptacle. The covers act as solar heat collectors and increase pile surface temperatures to above the thermal death point for fly eggs.

The ventpipe keeps the "gopuri" reasonably odourfree. The "sopa sandas", if equipped with a ventpipe, would be completely free of odours.

The receptacles should be large enough for a retention time of at least six months, preferably longer.

MEXICO: the solar heated, double-vault compost latrine

Following the publication of the preliminary edition of this book in 1978, a number of prototypes have been constructed in different countries. A solar heated compost latrine has been tried at a low-cost housing project in the town of Merida in southern Mexico.

This latrine works like a "gopuri" or "sopa sandas" unit. It has a seat riser place above a baffle between the two chambers. The baffle directs the input to one of the chambers. When that chamber is full, a handle is turned and the input falls into the other chamber.

A screened ventpipe extends from the receptacle to above the roof. One pipe serves both chambers. It ventilates away odours and also acts as a fly-trap as described on page 52.

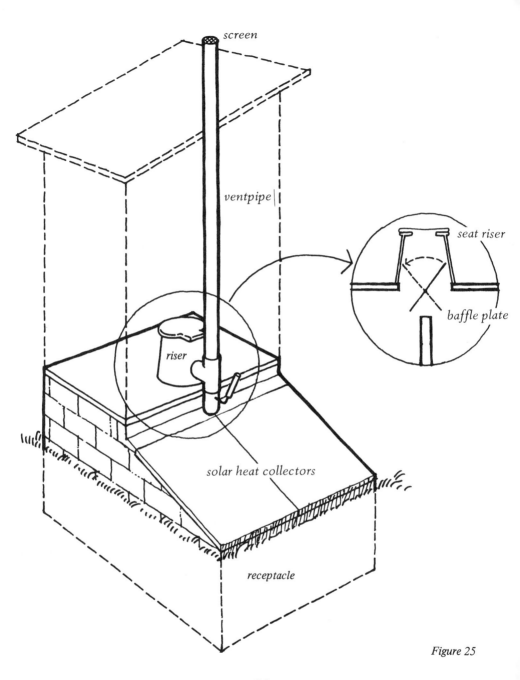

screen

ventpipe

seat riser

baffle plate

riser

solar heat collectors

receptacle

Figure 25

39

The chambers extend outside the superstructure and are covered with black painted lids made of aluminium sheets. The lids are facing south (north of the equator) and therefore act as solar heat collectors, increasing the evaporation from the receptacle as well as the surface temperature of the compost pile.

The chambers are only 0.75 m wide but over 2 m long. By shifting the pile to the rear end of the chamber with the help of a hoe, the capacity of the receptacle can be almost doubled. This means that the latrine has to be emptied only once a year at the most (if used regularly by 6 - 8 persons). The shifting of the pile to the rear end of the receptacle should be done when it is nearly full.

This latrine is more elaborate than the Indian types described on the previous pages and therefore more expensive to construct. It is, however, a permanent structure with a high capacity. The baffle makes the change from one chamber to the other an easy operation.

With a retention time of more than a year and an increased temperature due to the solar heater, this compost latrine should achieve a high degree of pathogen destruction.

SWEDEN: the "multrum" toilet

The "multrum" is a compost latrine consisting of a receptacle with a slanting floor, air conduits, and at the lower end a storage chamber. A tube connects the toilet seat with the receptacle and there is often a special chute for kitchen refuse.

A draft is maintained by natural convection from an air intake in the storage chamber, through the air conduits and out via a ventpipe. The ventpipe should reach at least 6 m above the toilet seat or garbage opening, whichever is higher. (Sometimes an exhaust fan is installed in the ventpipe.)

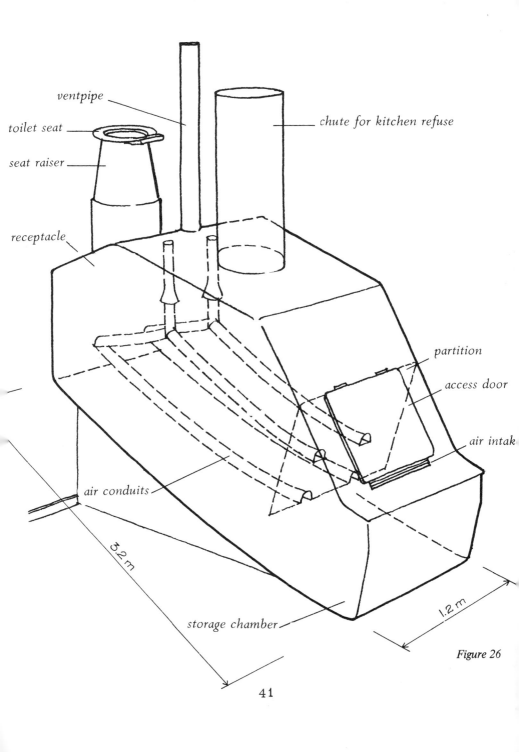

ventpipe

toilet seat

seat raiser

chute for kitchen refuse

receptacle

partition

access door

air intake

air conduits

3.2 m

1.2 m

storage chamber

Figure 26

41

The "multrum" was developed in Sweden about forty years ago. In the beginning it was made of concrete but is now usually put together from prefabricated parts made of fiberglass.

The inclined floor (slope about 30°) is covered with a starter bed consisting of a 0.4 m thick layer of peat moss and a 0.2 m layer of humus-rich garden soil (not raw subsoil or clay) mixed with grass cuttings. The purpose of this bed is to absorb liquid matter and to provide the microbes required for the oxidation of urine.

Into a "multrum" can go not only faeces and urine but all kinds of organic kitchen and household residues: vegetable and meat scraps, peelings, bones, eggshells, floor sweepings, sanitary napkins, and grass clippings. Cans, glass and plastic should not be put into a "multrum" and no large amounts of liquid of any kind. Any material which could get hung up on the air conduits and impede the settling of the pile should not be put in.

When the "multrum" is used, a compost heap is building up in the receptacle. Due to the slope of the floor the contents are slowly sliding from the fresh deposits at the upper end down to the storage chamber. In the meantime the decomposition process reduces the heap to less than 10% of the original volume.

The end product, a black, lumpy substance similar to good dry garden compost, accumulates at the lowest end of the inclined floor. This is a very slow process and the first time it may take four or five years until there is any need to remove humus from the storage chamber. After that a removal once a year should be sufficient. (The receptacle itself is never emptied. Only the material which has passed under the partition separating the storage chamber from the rest of the receptacle is removed.) The amount of humus produced varies from 10 to 30 litres per person per year.

The maximum number of users depends on factors such as temperature, humidity, amount and type of refuse, proportion of urine to faeces, and volume of the receptacle. In most cases 8 - 10 people would be the maximum for one "multrum" unit in regular, year round use.

42

The bacterial composition of the removed humus is similar to that of soil and in Sweden it is considered safe for use directly as a fertilizer and soil conditioner.

Various types of "multrum" are sold in the Scandinavian countries and now also in USA and Canada. The one illustrated here, the "Clivus multrum", is the largest one. It has a volume of 3 - 4 cu m and is usually installed in a basement directly under bathroom and kitchen.

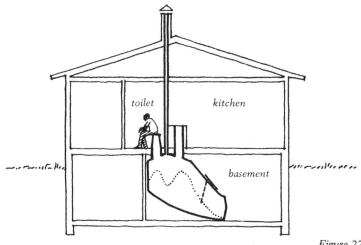

toilet   kitchen

basement

Figure 27

When used as a freestanding privy the "multrum" can be placed in a shallow pit and partly outside the building structure.

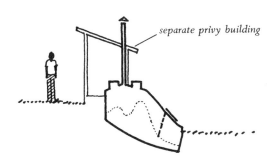

separate privy building

Figure 28

43

From an ecological point of view the "multrum" is the ideal solution. There is no contamination of soil or water. Carbon dioxide and water vapour constitute the major products released in the air. The end product is humus.

From a health point of view "multrum" units cannot be considered as safe as double-vault latrines. The reason for this is that pathogenic organisms can be washed from the top of the pile down to the storage chamber. (This cannot happen in a double-vault latrine as the two compartments are separated by a solid wall.) Fly breeding is another potential health hazard.

A correctly installed "multrum" is reasonably nuisance-free. When the unit is placed inside a house fruit-flies may cause a problem and on still, humid days there might be some odours. These problems would not be noticeable for a "multrum" placed in a separate shelter at some distance away from the dwelling house.

The cost of a prefabricated fibreglass "multrum" is far above what would be feasible in a developing country. Present prices in Scandinavia and North America range from US dollars 1600 to 2000, not including installation. A modified version of the "multrum" has been developed and tested in Tanzania and can be built from local material for a fraction of this cost. (Gurak, Kilama, and Winblad 1977)

YEMEN: the "long drop" latrine I

In the old part of the city of Sana as in other Yemenite towns the houses are slender and tall, rising five to nine storeys from narrow streets. A house is usually occupied by one extended family. Each floor has one or two lavatory-bathrooms located next to a vertical shaft extending from a receptacle at the street level to the uppermost bathroom as shown on the figure opposite.

The faeces drop via a hole in the squatting slab down the shaft to the receptacle from where they are collected at frequent intervals and brought to the public baths.

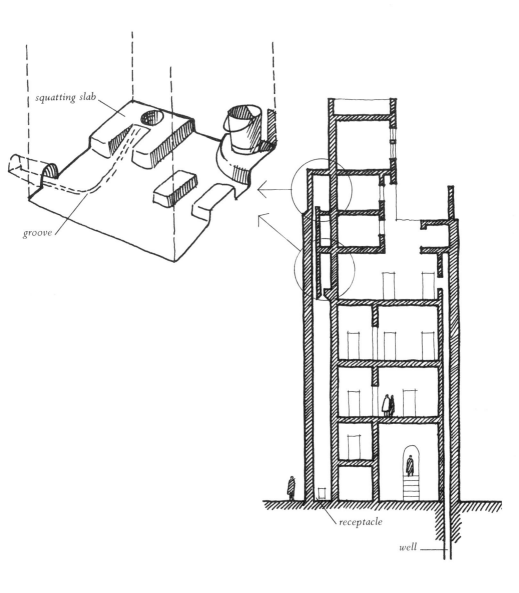

squatting slab

groove

receptacle

well

Figure 29

45

Sana has eighteen public baths, the oldest dating back to medieval times. The baths are used by almost everyone once a week. They are run by hereditary bath-keepers who charge a small fee for their use.

At the bathhouse the faeces are spread out on the roof to dry. Wood is scarce in Sana and the dried faeces are therefore used as fuel supplemented by the refuse of skins and bones from the slaughter yards. After burning, the ashes are sold as fertilizer for the orchards and vegetable gardens in town.

The urine is drained away from the squatting slab to a groove in the stone floor, from where it passes through an opening in the outside wall, to run down a vertical drainage surface on the outer face of the building. These drains are often elegantly shaped and decorated. As soon as it reaches the ground, the part of the liquid not evaporated on the way disappears into an underground drainage sump.

Anal cleansing takes place on a pair of square stones next to the squatting slab. The used water is drained away the same way as the urine. No liquids are thus led into the "long drop" shaft or the receptacle below. As Sana has a hot, dry climate the faeces quickly dehydrate which facilitates removal (Kirkman 1976, Lewcock 1976).

This system may seem odd but is indeed well adapted to the local situation: multi-storey buildings, extremely dry climate, scarcity of water and lack of firewood. Ecologically it is sound: There is no pollution of water or soil.

From the health point of view it would hardly be acceptable as it involves handling of fresh excreta. Whilst drying on the roof of the bath the faeces are accessible to flies. This need not be a problem though, as flies rarely lay eggs in any material with a moisture content of less than 65 %.

The final disposal of ashes is safe as burning efficiently destroys all pathogenic organisms.

46

ALGERIA: the single-vault compost latrine

In the town of Ouargla in the Algerian desert, environmental conditions are in some ways similar to those of Sana in Yemen. The climate is hot and dry, the housing density is high, streets are narrow and the whole town was until recently surrounded by a wall. Most houses are only two or three storeys high. The ground water table is extremely high and may reach within 0.3 m of the ground surface.

The traditional system of excreta disposal in Ouargla is compost latrines. The latrine is located inside the house and placed against a wall facing the street. It consists of a squatting slab above a shallow receptacle at or slightly below street level. From the latrine on the first floor there is a "long drop" chute to the same receptacle. In the receptacle the excreta are composted with palm leaves. It is emptied via an opening towards the street.

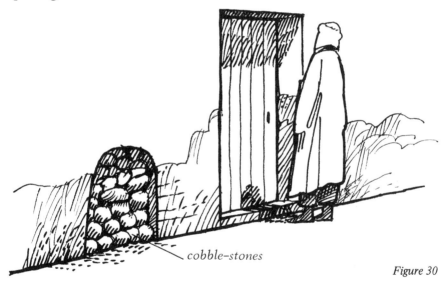

cobble-stones

Figure 30

The cobble-stones covering the hole in the wall are removed and the contents put in baskets and carried away. The compost is sold and used as a soil conditioner and fertilizer for date palm plantations outside the town wall (Asklund 1972).

The system described on the previous page is ecologically sound but doubtful from a health point of view. The weakness is that it is a single-vault latrine. When the receptacle is emptied, most of the contents are completely decomposed but there are also fresh excreta. To satisfy basic health criteria it is necessary to have two vaults or latrines used alternately.

W. GERMANY: the "long drop" latrine II

The "long drop" system has also been used in Europe according to a German handbook on masonry construction (Behringer 1959). Unlike the Yemenite system the German "long drop" latrine does not separate urine and faeces. The receptacle is water tight and dimensioned for an excreta volume of 500 litres per person per year. The contents have to be pumped out when the receptacle is full.

The German variation of the "long drop" system is less satisfactory than the Yemenite one as the contents of the receptacle will liquefy. The receptacle therefore has to be emptied by a vacuum truck or some other pumping device.

The reason for including it here is that with some modifications it could be turned into a compost system.

48

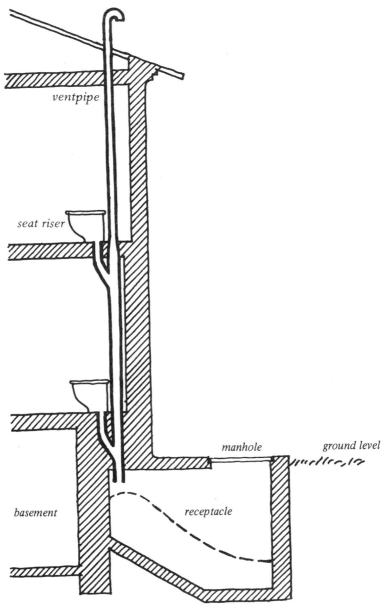

ventpipe

seat riser

manhole

ground level

basement

receptacle

Figure 31

49

TANZANIA: the traditional pit latrine

The pit latrine is used in many parts of the world. In its simplest form it consists of a large hand-dug pit covered with a squatting slab made of timber and soil as shown on the figures opposite.

In Tanzania the pit is often 1 m wide, 2 m long and 3-4 m deep. When it is full, another pit is dug nearby and a new shelter built on top. The shelter consists of a screen wall only. Usually there is no roof.

The input is excreta plus cleaning agent: water is used by Muslims and by most people along the coast and in other Muslim dominated areas. Banana and other leaves, grass, corncobs, paper etc are used in other parts of the country.

This simple form of latrine has important advantages: its function is readily understood and where soil and ground water conditions are right it is easy to construct from local resources.

The pit latrine also has serious weak points. It requires special ground conditions: the soil must be deep, stable and permeable, and the ground water table should be lower than the depth of the pit. These restrictions are often overlooked, resulting in pit collapse, especially when heavy rains have destabilized the soil, and in large scale mosquito breeding when liquid matter accumulates in the pit because of impermeable soil or high ground water table. The pit provides a protected breeding ground for filth flies and Culex mosquitoes, and the soil on the platform a hatching place for hookworms. The odours may be extremely offensive. The lifetime of the pit is often limited to a few years.

Under favourable circumstances the pit latrine can be an excellent solution to problems of excreta disposal. For instance at Omdurman in the Sudan there are latrines which have been in use from time immemorial. Some pits are over 20 m deep. But it is a rare exception. Frequently the traditional pit latrine is a health hazard and a nuisance.

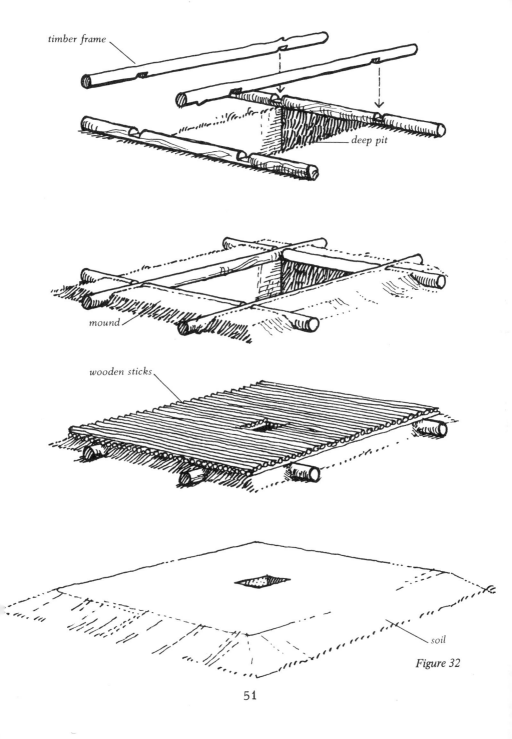

timber frame

deep pit

mound

wooden sticks

soil

Figure 32

51

ZIMBABWE: the ventilated pit latrine

Some of the shortcomings of the traditional pit latrine have been overcome by the "Blair Ventilated Privy", developed by the Blair Research Laboratory in Salisbury in the mid-70s. It consists of a squatting slab of reinforced concrete placed over a deep, partly lined pit. The slab has two openings: a squatting hole and a vent hole. The vent hole is outside the superstructure and fitted with a fluepipe, 150 mm in diameter and about 2.5 m high. The pipe should be painted black and be located on the sunny side of the superstructure. The upper part of the pipe is cone-shaped and opens out to 200 mm. The opening is covered with a copper or fiberglas flyscreen.

Temperature difference between the inside and the outside of the pipe will cause a convection updraught, drawing air and gases from the pit and thus causing a downdraught through the squatting hole. Flies from outside are attracted to the odours passing up the pipe and are said to avoid the interior of the superstructure. As the flies cannot enter the pit via the flue-pipe, fly-breeding in the pit is reduced. Flies breeding in the pit are attracted by the light at the top of the fluepipe and trapped there by the screen. Eventually they die there and fall back into the pit.

For the system to work, the superstructure must darken the squatting hole sufficiently for the flies inside the pit to be attracted by the light at the top of the fluepipe. The spiral shaped shelter without a door, see figure opposite, has been the most successful type in Zimbabwe. The walls are made of ferrocement (see page 91).

This improved latrine has several advantages over the traditional type. The pit is partly lined which might reduce the risk of pit collapse. The concrete slab can be cleaned and does not provide a breeding ground for hookworms. The fluepipe makes the latrine practically odour-free and reduces the fly nuisance.

Other deficiencies remain. The latrine cannot be built where the ground water table is high or the ground rocky. When the pit fills up, a new latrine has to be built. Culex mosquitoes will breed in the pit if it turns wet. In spite of the lining around the top of the pit, it might collapse. On the whole, however, the "Blair Ventilated Privy" is a considerable improvement over the traditional pit latrine.

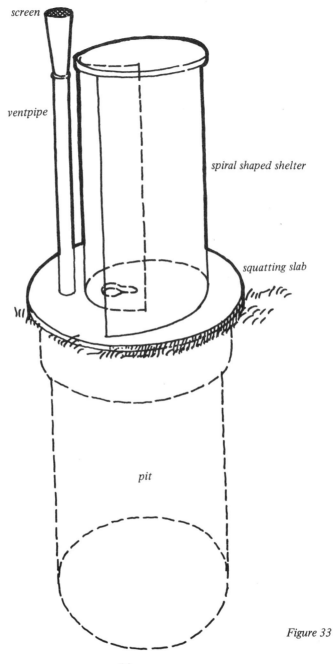

screen

ventpipe

spiral shaped shelter

squatting slab

pit

Figure 33

53

USA: the "earth-pit privy"

In 1933 the United States Public Health Services published a
handbook on latrine building called "The sanitary privy". It
claimed to include designs which represented the best sanitary
privy practices in the various States.

The "earth-pit privy" as recommended in the US almost fifty
years ago can be regarded as a luxury model of the traditional
pit latrine. The more subtle details of its construction are
eloquently described by Charles Sale (1929) in "The Specialist".

The receptacle is an excavated pit, 1 x 1 m square and at least
1.5 m deep. The pit is provided with a wooden curbing extending 0.15 - 0.20 m above the original ground line. The curbing
should cover the full depth of the pit unless the soil is very
stable, in which case the lower section of the curbing could be
omitted. The first three upper boards of the curb siding should
be tight. The lower boards may be spaced 20-30 mm apart.

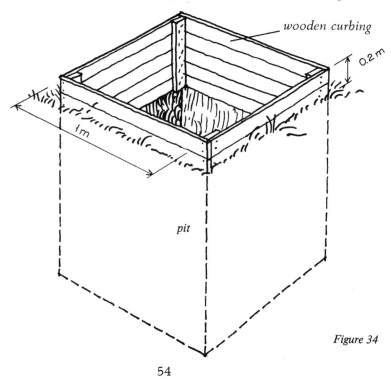

wooden curbing

0.2 m

1 m

pit

Figure 34

There must be a mound around the top of the curbing, sloping away from it to prevent surface water from entering the pit. The mound should extend for a distance of not less than 0.5 m and be level with the curbing. The soil of the mound should be rammed with a pice of solid timber as shown in the figure below.

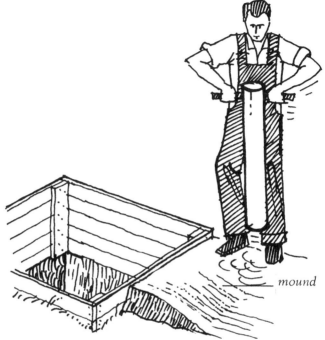

mound

Figure 35

Tongue-and-groove timber must be used for the platform and the seat riser to make them insect tight. Note in the illustration on the next page that the boards are placed vertically on the seat riser. This insures that urine is carried down into the pit and does not leak through, as might happen if the boards are laid horizontally.

A hinged lid and a ventpipe are fitted as shown in figure 36. (The hinges are made from strips cut out of the sidewalls of an old car tire.) The seat riser was often provided with two or more holes, frequently fashioned so as to accommodate persons of different sizes.

55

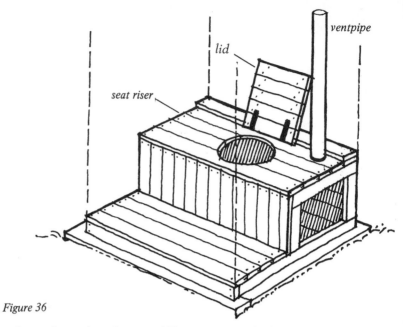

Figure 36

Compared to the traditional pit latrine of Tanzania type the "earth-pit privy" has the advantages of being non-collapsible due to the pit lining and less odorous due to the ventpipe. The other deficiencies remain. The raised seat has no advantage from a health point of view.

EGYPT: the borehole latrine

A variation of the borehole latrine was developed in S. E. Asia fifty years ago (Carter 1938), and has since been used in many countries including Egypt.

The receptacle is a vertical hole with a diameter of about 0.4 m and a depth of 6 m. It is bored in the ground with an auger as shown in the figure opposite. The wooden auger guide is not essential but simplifies the operations.

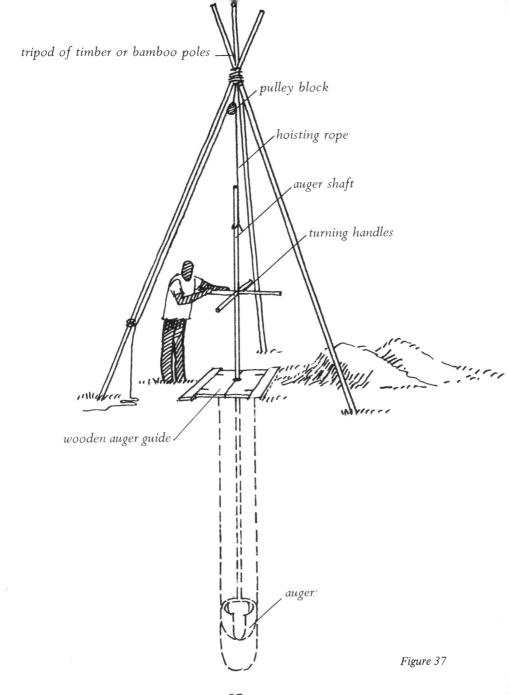

tripod of timber or bamboo poles

pulley block

hoisting rope

auger shaft

turning handles

wooden auger guide

auger

Figure 37

57

Around the top of the hole there is a collar of concrete or some other impervious material. Its purpose is to support the weight of the slab, to prevent the edges of the hole from caving and to prevent fly breeding in the earth under the slab.

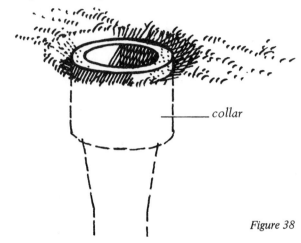

collar

Figure 38

The hole is covered with a squatting slab as shown in the figure below.

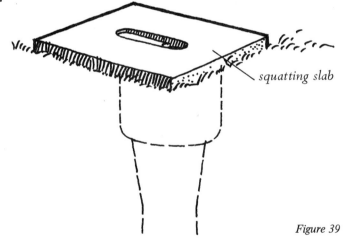

squatting slab

Figure 39

The auger should have a diameter of around 0.4 m. If much smaller, the side walls of the bored hole are easily fouled - if much larger, turning and emptying of the auger require considerably more power. Various types of augers can be used for digging borehole latrines.

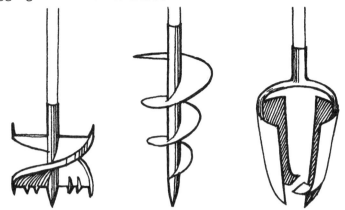

Figure 40

The subsoil must be sufficiently firm so that it will not cave in, yet soft enough to permit easy cutting by the auger. Caving is frequent with this type of latrine, especially in sandy or alluvial soils. In such cases it is necessary to provide the bored hole with a lining.

The lining should expose as large a part of the side walls as possible to the latrine contents as this contact plays an important role in the decomposition process.

A dry latrine 0.4 m wide and 6 m deep would fill up in less than two years if used regularly by 5 - 6 people. The life of a latrine reaching down into the ground water table can be much longer. In Egypt there are many that have been in regular use for more than eight years (Carter 1938).

The borehole latrine has much the same advantages and disadvantages as the ordinary pit latrine. Its lifetime is even shorter and it requires special construction equipment not usually available to individual households.

The "long-life" type with a wet borehole carries with it the risks of mosquito breeding and ground water pollution.

The often repeated statement that filth flies do not breed in deep, dark holes is not correct. Fly breeding can thus be a serious problem in this type of latrine.

S. AFRICA: Reid's Odourless Earth Closet

R.O.E.C. stands for Reid's Odourless Earth Closet and is a
type of improved pit latrine developed in S.Africa and patented
in 1944. The pit is 1 m wide, 2 m long and at least 3 m deep.
It is covered with a concrete slab and fitted with a 75 mm
diameter ventpipe. The squatting slab is on the side of the
receptacle as shown on the figure opposite.

The excreta are deposited in the pit via a chute. Only excreta
and toilet paper are deposited. The chute is not provided with
a lid.

The contents of the receptacle gradually decompose, liquids
are soaked up by the soil, and gases are ventilated away via
the ventpipe. Frech air is sucked down the chute.

Where soil conditions permit the liquid part of the excreta to
soak away, the pit fills up slowly. A receptacle with the
dimensions given above and with five to six regular users may
last for up to twenty years.

The R.O.E.C. can be attached to a house via a ventilated
passage and in some cases it is placed in the house (with the
pit outside the wall). This is possible as a properly constructed and well maintained R.O.E.C. unit is completely free
from odours.

An unlined pit should be dug with a slight inward slope towards
the bottom: 80 - 100 mm per metre depth is recommended. In
unstable soil the pit should be lined but holes must be provided
in the lining material to allow for soakage.

Around the top of the pit is a collar described in detail in
Chapter 5. The collar supports the cover slab of the receptacle. It is essential that the entire receptacle, collar and
cover slab are completely air tight and that the slab makes an
air tight joint on the collar of the pit. Any method of construction of this air tight cover slab may be used provided it is
strong enough.

In S.Africa some of the components are prefabricated in
asbestos cement: the ventpipe, the chute and the squatting

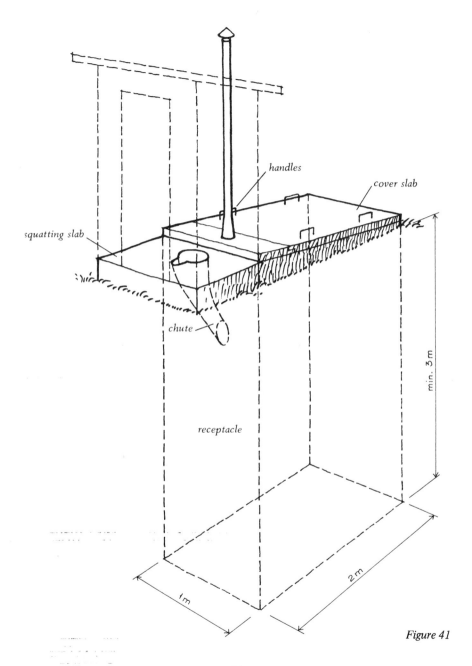

handles

cover slab

squatting slab

chute

receptacle

min. 3 m

1 m

2 m

Figure 41

61

slab (a pedestal seat is also available). The ventpipe can be made from any non-corrosive material as long as it is air tight. The chute can be made from a piece of drainpipe as shown in Chapter 4.

When a R.O.E.C. unit has been constructed, and before it is used for the first time, it should be tested for possible air leaks. A bundle of dry grass, newspapers or cotton waste soaked in oil is placed at the bottom of the receptacle, directly below the chute outlet. (This must be done before the cover slab is fitted over the pit.) When the installation is complete, the combustible material should be lit by dropping a piece of lighted paper down the chute. When the fire in the pit is burning properly, smoke will flow out of the top of the ventpipe, and a down draught can be noticed in the chute. Any smoke coming up the chute indicates a leak in the system. All leaks must be found and sealed. (Anon., no year.)

The ecological and health implications of a R. O. E. C. are the same as for a traditional pit latrine. The R. O. E. C. has some important advantages though: it is completely free from odours, the contents of the receptacle are not visible to the user of the latrine, there is no lid to replace, there is nothing to put in apart from the excreta and the latrine is not supposed to be emptied.

The patent holder's claim that the R. O. E. C. unit is "absolutely free from flies provided that no decomposed or other fly-blown matter is put into the pit" has not been verfied by tests carried out in Tanzania. Fly breeding is quite possible in a R. O. E. C. pit.

If liquids accumulate in the pit there is the additional possibility of mosquito breeding.

The chute makes it possible for rodents to move in and out of the receptacle.

As with all pit latrines, the risk of collapse is great, even with a lined pit.

The R. O. E. C. is probably the best version of the pit latrine. With some changes in construction and use it could be even better. (The construction of a modified R. O. E. C. unit is described in Chapter 5.)

REFERENCES CITED

ANONYMOUS (no year), *R. O. E. C. sanitation – installation instructions.* Bells Asbestoes & Engineering Africa Ltd, Johannesburg.

ASKLUND, L., JOHANSSON, S., KALNINS-NILSSON, A. & SELANDER, K. (1972), Ouargla – rapport från en algerisk ökenstad. Thesis (mimeo), Dept of Architecture, University of Lund, Lund, Sweden.

BEHRINGER, A. (1959), *Das Mauerbuch.* 9th ed. Otto Maier Verlag, Ravensburg, West Germany.

CARTER, J. C. (1938), The bored-hole latrine, Bull. Hyg. 13(8):591-599.

DEMOCRATIC REPUBLIC OF VIETNAM, Min. of Health, Dept of Hygiene and Epidemiology (1968), Double septic tanks, Hanoi, (mimeo).

DOROZYNSKI, A. (1975), When is waste a waste?, Ceres, **8** (5):70.

GURAK, R., KILAMA, W. & WINBLAD, U. (1977), Compost latrines in Tanzania - a preliminary report, Compost Science 18(4):20-23.

INDIA, CPHERI (1964), Evaluation of rural latrine designs, Proceedings of the Symposium, Nagpur.

KIRKMAN, J. (1976), *City of Sana,* World of Islam Publishing Co Ltd, London.

LEWCOCK, R. (1976), Towns and buildings in Arabia – N. Yemen, Arch. Ass. Quarterly 8(1):4-19.

McGARRY, M. & STAINFORTH, J. ed. (1978), *Compost fertilizer and biogas production from human and farm wastes in the People's Republic of China.* IDRC, Ottawa.

McMICHAEL, J. K. ed. (1976), *Health in the third world – studies from Vietnam,* Spokesman Books, Nottingham.

MORGAN, P. R. (1979), A ventilated pit privy, Appropriate Technology 6(3):10-11.

SALE, C. (1929), *The specialist,* Specialist Publishing Co, Carmel, Calif., USA.

UNITED STATES, Treasury Dept, Public Health Service (1933), *The sanitary privy,* Supplement No 108 to the Public Health Reports, Government Printing Office, Washington D.C.

FURTHER READING

WAGNER, E. G. & LANOIX, J. N. (1958), *Excreta disposal for rural areas and small communities,* WHO Monograph Series No 39, Geneva.

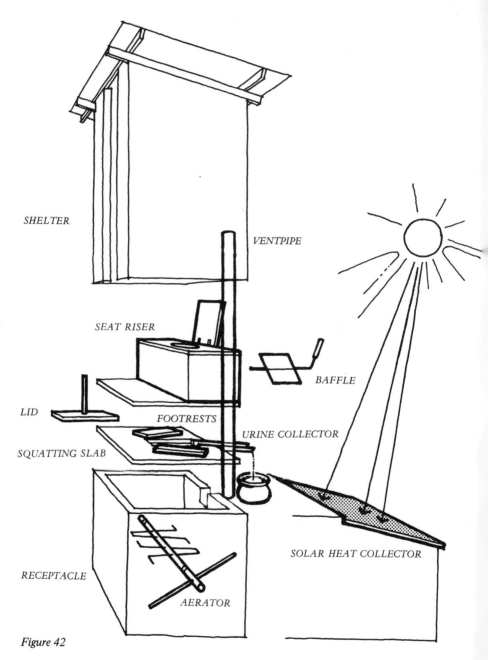

SHELTER

VENTPIPE

SEAT RISER

BAFFLE

LID

FOOTRESTS

URINE COLLECTOR

SQUATTING SLAB

SOLAR HEAT COLLECTOR

RECEPTACLE

AERATOR

Figure 42

64

Chapter 4

LATRINE COMPONENTS

The examples in Chapter 3 demonstrated the variety of established technical solutions to problems of sanitation without water. In this chapter we shall look at the technical components of a latrine system. In the following chapter we shall show you how to combine the components into latrines to fit specific local conditions.

The basic components of a latrine are the receptacle, squatting slab, lid and shelter. The "basic latrine" can be fitted with one or more optional components like ventpipe, aerator, footrests, seat riser, baffle plate, urine collector, and solar heat collector (see figure opposite).

RECEPTACLE

The function of the receptacle is to receive and safely store the excreta and what else is supposed to be placed in it.

Size and shape can vary considerably from one type of latrine to another. It can be very small, like the Chinese one described in the previous chapter. Such a receptacle has to be emptied daily and the excreta transferred to a compost heap. The system may be acceptable in China and Japan where there is an age old tradition of handling excreta this way, but in the rest of the world there is no reason to introduce it. Better systems are available.

The range of receptacles we can choose from is illustrated on the following page.

A shallow receptacle (double-vault, off-set double-vault, and long drop) serves as a temporary depository of excreta and often also of organic kitchen and garden residues. It has to be emptied at intervals determined by the number of users, the

65

SHALLOW RECEPTACLES

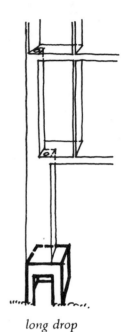

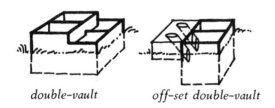

double-vault　　　*off-set double-vault*　　　*long drop*

DEEP RECEPTACLES

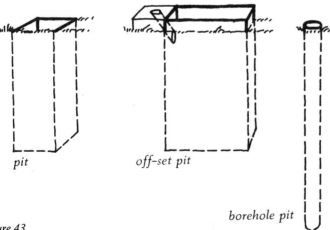

pit　　　*off-set pit*

borehole pit

Figure 43

66

nature of the input and the volume of the receptacle.

The shallow receptacle can be constructed as a closed vault, without any infiltration of liquids into the soil or as an open vault, that is, with a bottom formed by the subsoil.

The double-vault receptacle illustrated here is a development of the Indian "gopuri" and the Vietnamese type. This version can be emptied from above via a removable cover, which means that the receptacle can be placed as low as the ground water level permits.

The off-set double-vault receptacle is used in the Indian "sopa sandas" latrine. It is a type that can be easily fitted with flap-traps and/or a solar heat collector.

The long drop latrine is the one traditionally used in Yemen.

A deep receptacle (traditional pit, off-set pit, and borehole) serves as the final depository of the excreta. The traditional pit and the off-set pit should be at least 3 m deep in order not to fill up too fast. The borehole is usually taken to a depth of 6 m.

The bottom of the pit must in all cases be well above the highest ground water table to avoid creating favourable conditions for the breeding of *Culex* mosquitoes or pollution of drinking water supplies.

The traditional pit is the most common form of receptacle. Its advantages and drawbacks were described in the previous chapter under Tanzania. The off-set pit is used in the R.O.E.C. type of latrine described under S.Africa. The narrow and deep bore hole can only be dug with special equipment.

In its simplest form the receptacle consists of a hand-dug, unlined hole in the ground. To prevent the edges of the pit from collapsing they must be strengthened with a frame which should be placed in position before the pit is dug. The frame can be made from timber as in figure 32, or from reinforced concrete as in the figure at the top of the following page.

In unstable soil it is necessary to line the entire pit. Lining

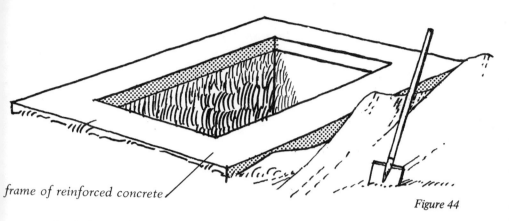

frame of reinforced concrete

Figure 44

material can be timber, stones or building blocks. If the lining reaches all the way down, the lower half must have open joints so that liquids can infiltrate the soil.

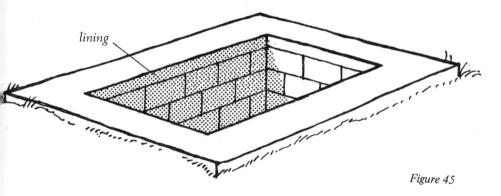

lining

Figure 45

The shallow receptacles are usually built as masonry vaults. They can be made from stones or any kind of building blocks: sundried bricks, soilcement blocks, concrete blocks or burnt bricks can be used. Where hardwood is available it is also possible to make the vault from timber.

It is not necessary to make the walls water-tight, but they have to be tight enough to prevent insects and rodents from getting in or out. They must also be strong enough to carry the squatting slab, the user and the superstructure.

68

If concrete blocks are made they need not, for a shallow receptacle, be more than 50 mm thick. Sixty blocks 50 x 190 x 390 mm can be made out of one 50 kg bag of cement.

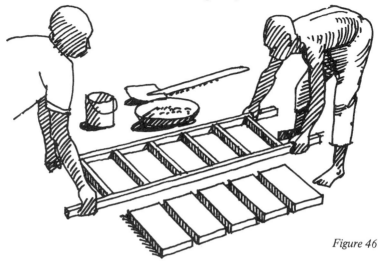

Figure 46

If a deep receptacle is to be lined it is necessary to use blocks with a thickness of 100-150 mm.

A concrete floor is not necessary if the receptacle is placed in a pit (unless there are domestic water wells nearby). Some polluted liquid may leak into the soil, but only under the most unusual circumstances will pathogenic organisms travel through more than a few metres of soil. If the receptacle is on or above the ground surface or the soil conditions are such that ground water pollution is possible, then it is advisable to have a concrete floor. (A watertight floor means that the amount of liquid that can go into the receptacle must be strictly limited. Separation of urine may be necessary, see figure 61.)

SQUATTING SLAB

The squatting slab can be placed either on top of the receptacle or outside it. In the first case the size and shape of the slab is determined by the receptacle.

The slab must have a hole, large enough to admit faeces and urine without the edges being soiled, small enough for children not to fall in.

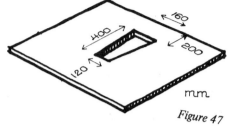

Figure 47

The slab must have a hard, smooth, easy-to-clean surface. A suitable material is ferrocement: a rich cement mortar reinforced with chicken wire. Reinforced concrete is commonly used, but such a slab is much too heavy for one man to to carry and costs more. A ferrocement slab 0.9 x 0.9 m need not be more than 18 mm thick and weighs about 35 kg. In Chapter 5 there is a detailed description of how to make a ferrocement slab.

The slab can be made from timber and earth as shown in figure 32. This is the most common construction in rural areas. The trouble with such a platform is that the soil surface cannot be properly cleaned and may turn into a breeding ground for parasites like hookworms and *Strongyloides stercoralis.* The timber support is often attacked by termites.

If the squatting slab is placed off-side the receptacle a chute is necessary. It can be made out of a piece of drainpipe or directly from ferrocement.

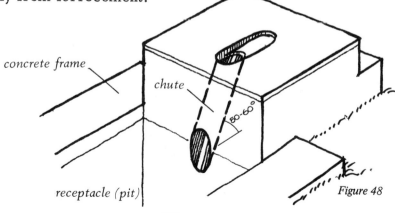

Figure 48

70

A diameter of 150 mm and a slope of 50°- 60° is what we re-
commend for the chute.

A squatting slab with a chute has some advantages: the contents of the receptacle are not visible and the chute can quite
easily be fitted with a self-closing lid, as shown in figure 52.
Experience has proved that the chute is virtually self-cleaning.

LID

The main purpose of a lid is to prevent insects and rodents
from moving in and out of the receptacle. A lid can be made
of wood.

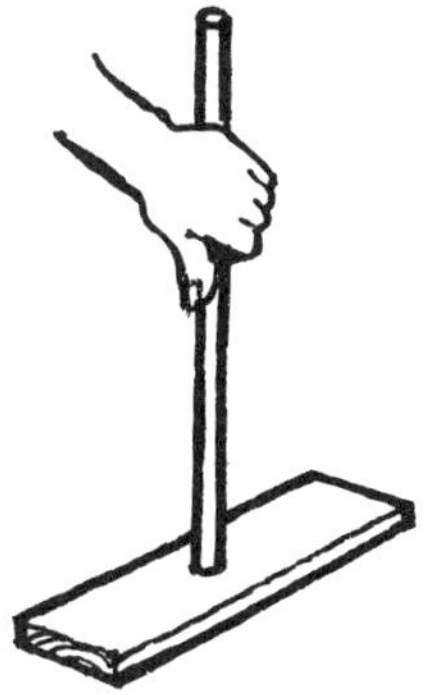

Figure 49

Double-vault latrines must have two lids. The one covering
the vault in use should be made from wood according to the
picture above. The lid for the other hole should be heavy and
difficult to remove to prevent the simultaneous use of both
vaults.

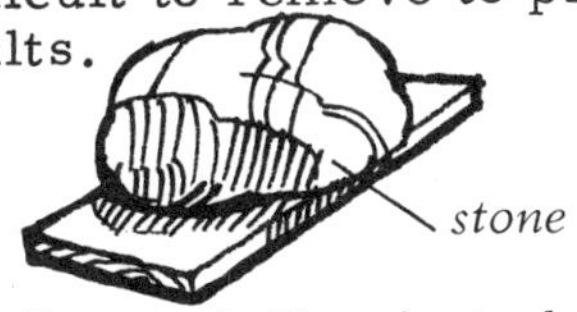

stone

Figure 50

Another solution is to have movable squatting slabs, one with
a hole, the other one without, see figure 21. This arrangement ensures that only one receptacle at a time can be used.

Seat risers are often provided with a hinged lid. This makes
sure that it is replaced correctly (if replaced at all). The
underside of the lid tends to be slimy and is certainly nothing
you want to lean your back against. From this point of view
it is better with a completely removable lid.

71

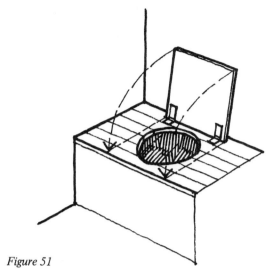

Figure 51

With a manually operated lid there is always the risk that it
is not replaced properly. This is a common experience from
latrine programmes all over the world. The lid ought to be
self closing. This is not so easy to fix unless the latrine has
a chute. The lower end of the chute can be provided with a
flap-trap consisting of a piece of tin suspended on two hooks
(use non-corroding metal). Occasionally some dirt may
prevent the tin flap from closing completely but like the chute
it is self-cleaning. The device has been tested on some
latrines in Tanzania and works very well indeed.

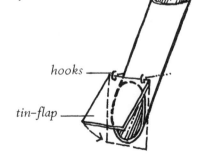

hooks

tin-flap

Figure 52

A squatting slab placed directly over the receptacle can only
be fitted with a flap-trap if the chute is provided first. A
chute can be shaped as part of the ferrocement slab as shown

72

in this figure. *pieces of wood for hinges*

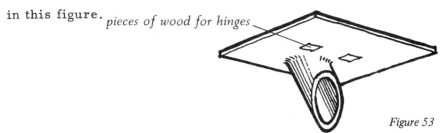

Figure 53

A tin flap is then attached as shown in figure 52. Two small pieces of wood have been incorporated into the slab above to facilitate the fixing of the hooks acting as hinges. An alternative to shaping the chute in ferrocement is to cast a short piece of drainpipe into the slab.

Another solution is to incorporate hole, chute and flap-trap into one prefabricated unit. This device is then placed upside down in the form used for casting the squatting slab and incorporated into the slab.

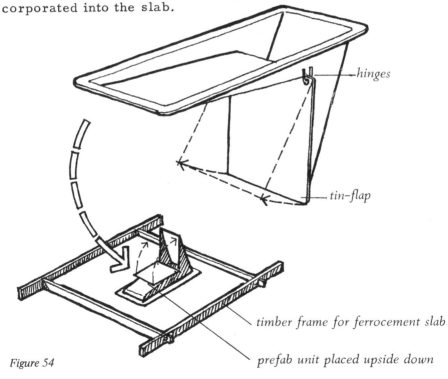

hinges

tin-flap

timber frame for ferrocement slab

Figure 54

prefab unit placed upside down

SHELTER

The purpose of the shelter, or superstructure, is to provide privacy and protection for the user and to prevent sunlight and rainwater from entering the receptacle. The last point is specially important for compost latrines as they must be kept dry. The superstructure should therefore be of sound construction and have a proper roof. Building blocks of the same kind as in the receptacle can be used.

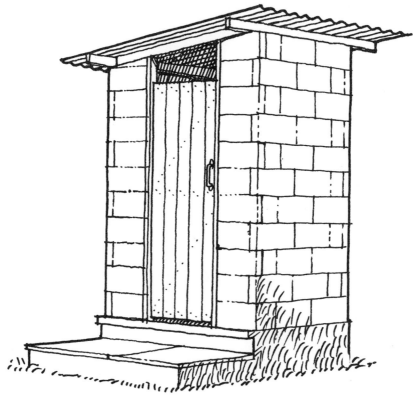

Figure 55

Traditional construction can be used - the important thing is that the structure must keep out rain.

74

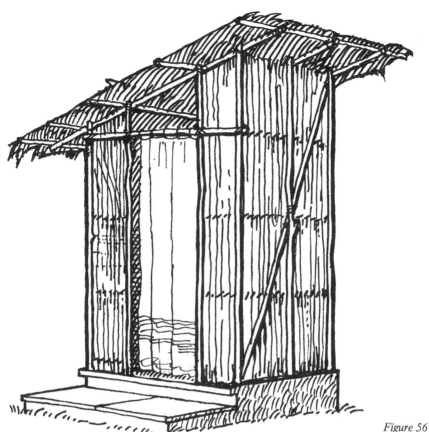

Figure 56

OPTIONAL COMPONENTS

Ventpipe

A ventpipe or flue is not necessary but improves the latrine in two important ways: odours are ventilated away and filth flies are trapped. The ventpipe can be made from bamboo, timber, masonry, ferrocement or plastic. A diameter of 150 mm would be about right. If the walls of the shelter are of masonry construction ventilation can be via a flue shaped by the building blocks.

The ventpipe opening at the top must be screened to prevent insects from getting in and out of the receptacle that way.

Copper mesh is preferable but ordinary nylon mosquito screens could be used. The wire mesh must be rustproof as the fumes from the latrine are highly corrosive.

The ventpipe should be painted black and be located on the sunny side of the latrine in order to increase the airflow through the pipe.

Aerator

The purpose of an aerator is to bring the interior of the pile in the receptacle into contact with the oxygen in the air. This can be achieved in a number of ways: by turning the pile, by bringing air conduits through it (see Chapter 3: China) and by adding large amounts of grass and straw. For a household size compost latrine turning is not necessary nor are air conduits essential. Most important is to add grass and straw to prevent the compost pile from turning compact and soggy.

Turning is, however, an efficient way of quickening the decomposition process. A simple turning device can be made from a length of galvanized pipe and a few pieces of reinforcement bars. The figure below illustrates the arrangement.

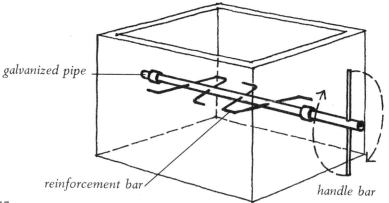

galvanized pipe

reinforcement bar

handle bar

Figure 57

Half a turn two or three times a week should be enough if the pile has the right moisture content. If the contents are wet the pile must be turned over once a day.

Footrests

The main purpose of the footrests is to guide the latrine user
in aiming right, particularly at night.

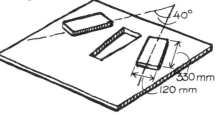

Figure 58

Seat riser

A raised seat is probably more convenient than a squatting
slab but is neither healthful nor hygienic. "The high toilet
seat may prevent complete evacuation. The natural position
for defecation ... is the squatting position ... When the thighs
are pressed against the abdominal muscles in this position,
the pressure within the abdomen is greatly increased, so that
the rectum is more completely emptied." (Kern 1970)

If for cultural reasons a squatting slab is not acceptable, a
seat riser can be added. It can be made from wood as in
figure 36 or from plastic as in figure 25.

In cultures where water is used for anal cleansing seat risers
should not be used as the cleansing water inevitably fouls the
seat.

Baffle plate

One advantage with a seat riser is that it gives the extra
space we need to fit the latrine with a baffle plate. Most
compost latrines have two squatting holes or a seat riser
with two holes. By using a baffle we need only one hole placed
above the partition dividing the receptacle into two chambers.

77

The baffle plate directs the latrine input (excreta and refuse) to one of the chambers. When that chamber is full, the baffle plate is turned via a handle. The input then falls into the other chamber.

Figure 59

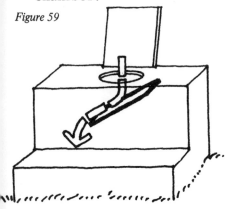 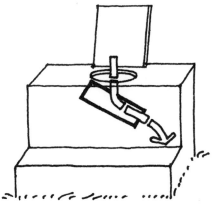

A latrine without a seat riser can be equipped with a baffle if the squatting slab is raised about 0.25 m.

Figure 60

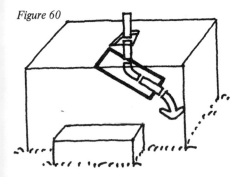 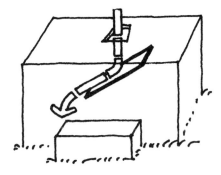

Urine collector

A latrine can be designed in such a way that the urine is collected separately and only the faeces are deposited in the

78

receptacle as shown by the examples from China, Vietnam
and Yemen in Chapter 3 of this book.

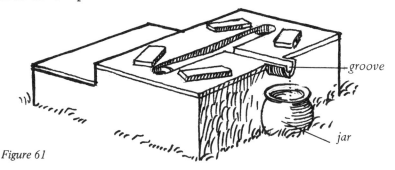

Figure 61

There are three reasons for separating the urine: to keep the
latrine contents dry, to reduce the need for adding high carbon
material (see section on carbon/nitrogen ratio in Chapter 2)
and to conserve the urine's fertilizer value. (The urine,
diluted with 5 parts of water, can be used in the vegetable
garden right away.)

In some cases it may be desirable to keep urine out of the
receptacle although for cultural reasons it cannot be used as
a fertilizer. Instead of collecting the urine in a jar, it can
be piped directly into a soakpit.

Solar heater

The temperature inside a receptacle can be increased if it is
designed and placed in such a way that parts of it are heated
by the sun. The temperature of the surface of the compost
heap can be augmented that way. The increase is likely to be
marginal but can be of importance in fly control as discussed
in the Appendix.

The easiest way of adding direct solar energy to the heat
generated by the decomposition process is to expose the upper
part of the receptacle to the sun and turn the cover into a
collector. It could, for instance, be made of a blackened
piece of aluminium sheet or ferrocement.

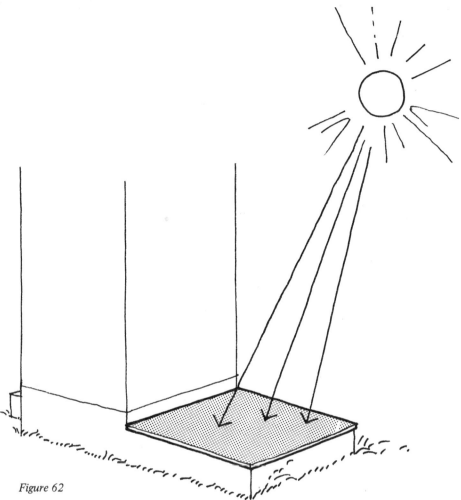

Figure 62

More elaborate systems incorporating collectors with glass cover and insulation material are outside the scope of this book.

REFERENCES CITED

KERN, K. (1970), *The owner-built home,* Specialty Printing Co, Yellow Springs, Ohio, p 66.

Chapter 5

HOW TO BUILD

The components described in the previous chapter can be combined in numerous ways. The final choice must depend on the local situation. Factors like climate, soil stability and permeability, ground water level, housing density, water supply, existing latrine habits, agricultural practices, motivation, building skills, building materials and money availability must be taken into consideration. The choice should be made by the prospective users once they have become aware of the range of alternatives and their implications.

We start this chapter with a brief discussion of the most important factors influencing the choice of latrine type, cost and location. The major part of the chapter shows in detail how to build four different types of latrines for individual households and also how to attach a simple "bathroom". At the end of the chapter there is an example of how a latrine type illustrated in this book can be adapted to institutional use.

SELECTION

In selecting a latrine type for a specific location the first choice should be between a compost system and a final deposit system. The former usually includes a shallow receptacle while the latter generally relies on a deep receptacle or pit.

A compost system should be your choice

> if the subsoil makes the digging of a deep pit impossible or extremely difficult,

> if the ground water sometimes comes within 3 m of the ground surface,

> if you want to utilize the decomposed excreta as a soil conditioner and fertilizer.

A compost system in this context most often means a double-

vault latrine with the squatting slab directly on top of the receptacle. The Vietnamese type and the "gopuri" latrine from India
are typical examples. This chapter contains a step-by-step
description of how to build such a latrine. For those who prefer
an off-set double-vault type we have added a description of a
slightly modified version of the Indian "sopa sandas".

The double-vault latrine   The off-set double-vault latrine

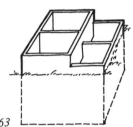
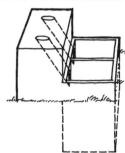

Figure 63

A final deposit system is likely to be your choice

> if handling and reuse of decomposed excreta is
> unacceptable, provided it is possible to dig a
> deep pit, and you are sure the ground water
> never comes within 3 m of the ground surface.

A final deposit system means some kind of pit latrine. In this
chapter we are describing two types: the ventilated pit latrine
and the modified R.O.E.C. latrine.

The ventilated pit latrine   The modified R.O.E.C.

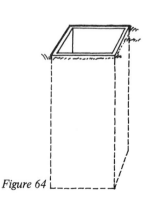
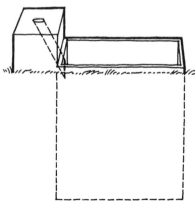

Figure 64

We have added a brief description of a multi-unit compost latrine suitable for institutions.

COSTS

Expected expenses for materials and construction will no doubt influence your choice but we have not included cost estimates in this book. The reason is that building costs expressed in monetary terms can be completely misleading. The real cost depends on who is building (the owner himself, local artisans or a building contractor), how many units are to be produced (repetition makes for economy in formwork and skills), and on the extent to which local materials can be used.

The monetary costs can vary from virtually nil if only locally available resources are used to over a thousand dollars if a contractor is going to do the job with hired labour and pre-fabricated components. The two extremes are illustrated in Chapter 3 by the examples from Vietnam (entirely self-built, no material purchased) and Sweden (prefabricated unit sold at a price equivalent of US dollars 1600 - 2000).

The first compost latrine illustrated on the following pages can be built by two people in about a week. Two and a half 50 kg bags of cement are required for making 150 concrete blocks 50 x 190 x 390 mm. Another bag of cement is required for mortar and for the ferrocement slabs. About 6 sq m of chicken-wire mesh is necessary as reinforcement of slabs and covers. The rest of the job could be done with locally available materials: sand, timber poles, grass, reeds, coconut leaves or banana leaves.

Three bags of cement and 6 sq m chicken-wire mesh are required for the modified R.O.E.C. unit described later on in this chapter. Only 25 concrete blocks (50 x 190 x 390 mm) are used. Most of the cement is required for the pit frame and the ferrocement covers. Other materials to be purchased include 12 m reinforcement bars, two hooks for the flap-trap and a 1 m piece of 150 mm drainpipe for the chute. What else is required for the construction should be available locally. (If the soil is unstable and the whole pit has to be lined 225 concrete blocks of 100 - 150 mm thickness are required.)

LOCATION

The choice of latrine type can be influenced by the water supply system in the vicinity of the proposed latrine location. If the latrine is to be built near a well the following factors must be considered: type of latrine, ground water level, slope of the ground, and subsoil conditions.

A latrine with a tight receptacle from which there is no filtration does not pollute the ground water. With filtration the risk of ground water pollution is virtually nil if the bottom of the receptacle is more than 1.5 m above the ground water table and the soil is uniform and free from cracks. If the bottom of the receptacle is close to or reaches down into the ground water, the latrine must be located downhill from the well. This is due to the fact that contamination does not move against the direction of flow of the ground water. Where uphill locations cannot be avoided, a distance of 15 m will prevent bacterial pollution of the well. In sandy soil a latrine may be placed as close as 7.5 m from a properly constructed household well if it is impossible to place it at a greater distance (Wagner and Lanoix 1958).

In areas containing fissured rocks or limestone formations seepage from the latrine can be carried long distances. For such conditions it is essential that the latrine is placed downhill from the well.

The distance required between a latrine and a dwelling is determined by the type of latrine and the housing density (plot size) as well as by considerations of convenience and nuisance.

At low housing densities (large plot sizes) most people would probably place their latrine at a distance of 10 - 20 m from the dwelling. A longer distance may mitigate against regular use and proper maintenance of the latrine, and there is also the risk that it will be misused by passers-by not belonging to the household. In crowded urban conditions there is no choice. The latrine has to be placed close to or even inside the dwelling. Odours need not be a problem if the latrine has a ventilated receptacle. More difficult is the problem of insects attracted to or breeding inside the latrine. Most latrines in the tropics are full of cockroaches (as are most septic tanks).

84

As long as they stay inside the receptacle their presence is beneficial as they contribute to the decomposition process but they are not wanted in the dwelling, especially not in the kitchen. Cockroaches are virtually impossible to get rid of and very difficult to contain. From this point of view, therefore, the greater the distance between latrine and kitchen, the better.

Under crowded conditions a compost latrine would be a better choice than a pit latrine. First because the compost latrine is a permanent installation. Second, there is no need for a deep pit which could destabilize the foundations of nearby houses. Third, there is no infiltration of liquid into the soil.

COMPOST SYSTEMS
The double-vault latrine

The double-vault latrine is a compact, versatile unit suitable wherever people accept the idea of composting human excreta. The basic structure shown here (figures 67-73) can be varied in a number of ways and with some ingenuity it could be fitted with a selection of optional components described in the previous chapter. Several units can be combined into one multi-unit as shown at the end of this chapter. (If you want a flap-trap and a solar heater on your latrine, the off-set double-vault receptacle should be selected, see figures 75-76.)

If the area where you are building your latrine is flat and waterlogged you should place it on a mound and provide the receptacle with a watertight floor as in Vietnam (see figure 65 on the next page).

If the ground water never reaches within a metre or two of the surface of the ground you may place the receptacle in a pit. Then there is usually no need for a watertight floor. The unit we are illustrating on the following pages consists of two vaults each 1.3 m by 0.8 m (internal measurements) and at the most 1.2 m high. The walls are made from concrete blocks 50, 75 or 100 mm thick, 190 mm high and 390 mm long.

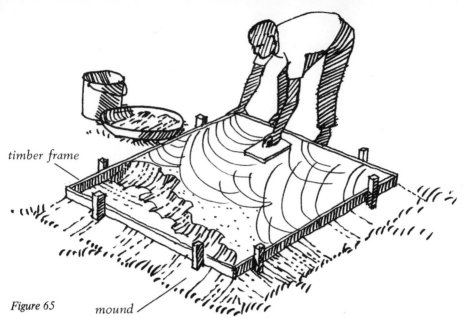

timber frame

Figure 65   mound

Start by digging a pit approximately 1.5 x 1.8 m. The pit could
be up to 1.0 m deep depending on the location of the highest
ground water table. In the series of illustrations that follows
we have indicated the pit as being 0.5 m deep. The earth floor
of the pit is also the bottom of the receptacle.

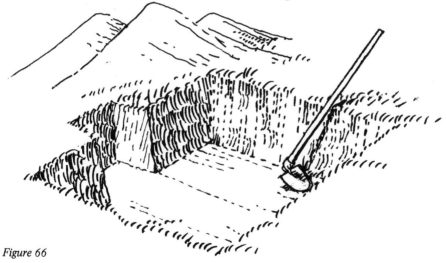

Figure 66

86

For the first four layers (0.8 m) you just take the five walls straight up. The receptacle is divided into two vaults by a partition as shown below.

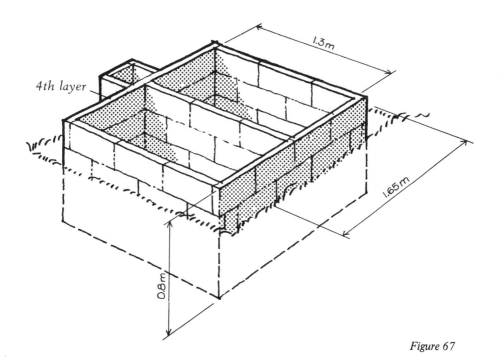

Figure 67

The fifth layer is laid the same way but here you put some blocks across to provide a beam. Place this beam 0.8m from the rear wall. The blocks forming the beam must be supported until the mortar has set. The span is so short that there is no need for any permanent reinforcement.

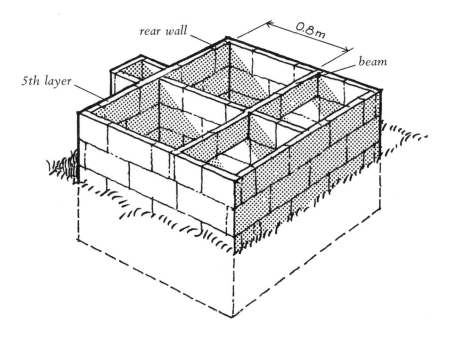

Figure 68

If you are using 50 mm blocks: before you proceed with the sixth layer, put some blocks on the flat side around the front part of the receptacle as shown by the figure below. These blocks provide support for the covers to be added later.

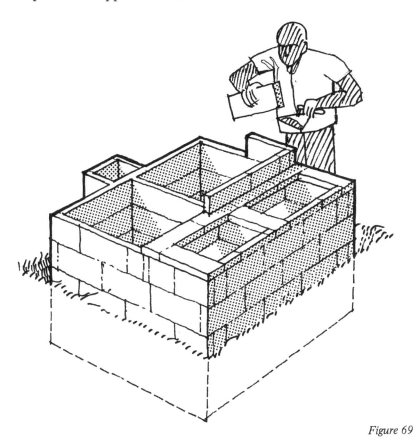

Figure 69

The sixth layer is placed only around the part of the receptacle to be covered by the squatting slab. Leave a hole for the flue.

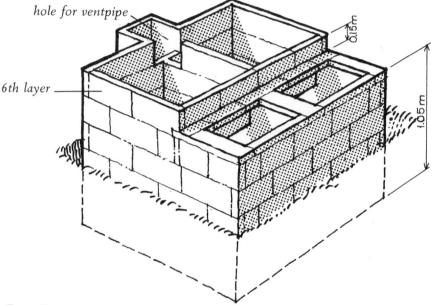

Figure 70

Before you continue the masonry work, the squatting slabs must be placed in position.

Squatting slabs and covers are best made from ferrocement. This is a mixture of cement, sand and water reinforced with chicken-wire mesh. Make a form for the squatting slab: internal measurements 0.9 x 0.87 m and 18 mm deep. (The slab need not be more than 18 mm thick!) Place three layers of chicken-wire mesh in the form. Cut out the hole, 0.12 x 0.40 m through the three layers and place a block of wood there. (If wire mesh is not available it is possible to reinforce the slab with sisal fibre or coconut fibre.)

90

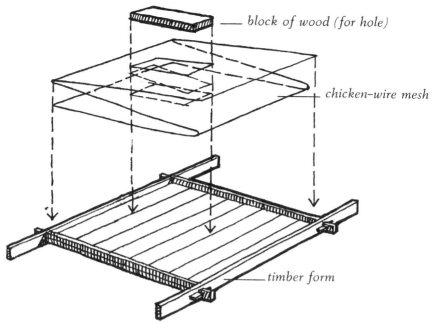

block of wood (for hole)

chicken-wire mesh

timber form

Figure 71

Mix one part cement with two parts sand. For a slab of 0.9 x 0.9 m and 18 mm thick you need 11 kg (9.5 litres) cement and 22 kg (17.5 litres) sand. Add water until you have a r ather stiff mortar (roughly 0.4 part water by weight). Too much water in the mortar will reduce the strength of the slab.

Apply the mortar with a trovel and force it into the layers of mesh. Press the mortar hard and shake the form by tapping it with a hammer so that no empty spaces will be left inside the slab.

Place the form with the slab in the shade and cover it with wet sacking to prevent the slab from drying out during the cement hardening process. Keep the sacks wet.

After 24 hours the slab can be taken out of the form and the form used again. Put the slab in the shade for a few days and keep it covered with wet sacks.

Footrests can be moulded in cement mortar. If slabs are
to be massproduced it is better to incorporate the shape of
the footrests in the form for the slab.

The process is repeated for the second slab and the two covers
are made in the same way. Make the covers 0.50 x 0.87 m and
about 18 mm thick. They should preferably be made with a
rim (see figure 76) to make it more difficult for the flies to
escape through the joint between the covers and the receptacle.
The figure below shows the squatting slab and the covers in
position. The squatting slabs are placed permanently and
should be set in mortar while the covers must be removable.

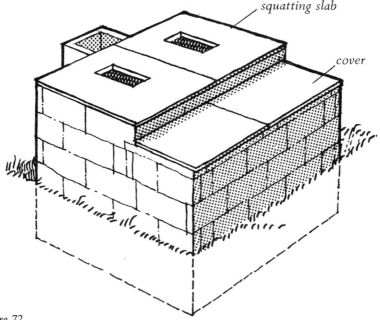

squatting slab

cover

Figure 72

Continue the masonry work until the superstructure, including the fluepipe, is completed. Add steps, door, roof
and, on top of the flue, a mosquito screen.

Put several layers of well tampered earth against the walls
of the receptacle so that rain water is drained away from
the latrine.

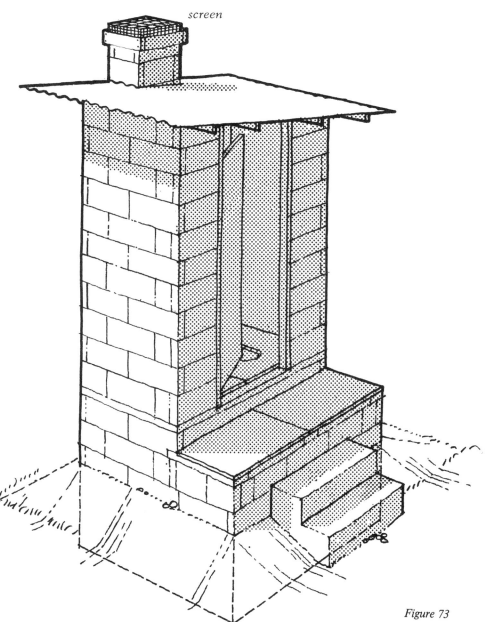

screen

Figure 73

Before the latrine is used it must be provided with lids for the holes in the double squatting slab, see figures 49 and 50.

The off-set double-vault latrine (modified "sopa sandas")

If you want a compost latrine with a flap-trap and a solar
heat collector you should, as mentioned previously, start
with an off-set double-vault receptacle.

This type can also be placed entirely above ground if necessary. However, the distance from the bottom of the receptacle to the top of the squatting slab is nearly two metres so
it is better if you can place at least half of the receptacle
underground. The unit illustrated here consists of two vaults
0.8 x 0.8 m internally. The total height of the receptacle
should be at least 1.2 m. You can increase the height up to
1.8 m if you want a receptacle with a greater capacity. If you
make it higher it might be difficult for you to empty the receptacle.

Start by digging a pit approximately 1.0 x 2.0 m. The depth of
the pit should be about 0.2 m less than the total height of the
receptacle (if the ground water level permits!). In the figure
below we have indicated the pit as being 0.8 m deep. The earth
floor of the pit forms the bottom of the receptacle.

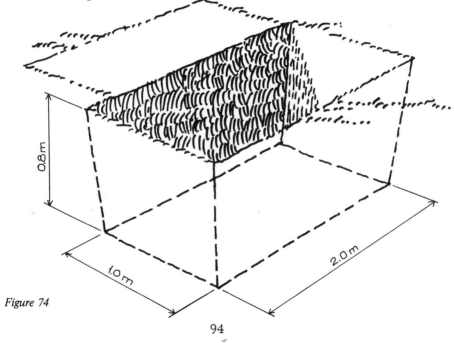

0.8 m

1.0 m

2.0 m

Figure 74

94

The masonry work for the receptacle is apparent from the figure below.

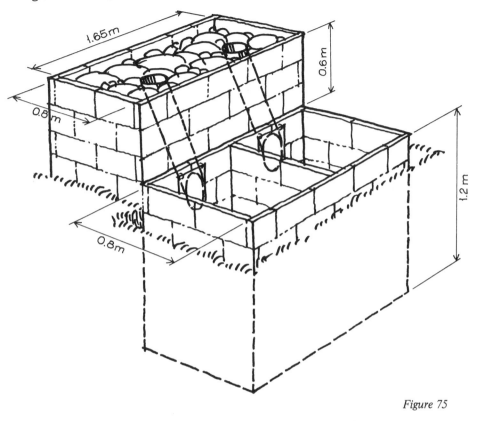

1.65 m

0.8 m

0.6 m

0.8 m

1.2 m

Figure 75

The squatting slab is placed 0.6 m above the top of the receptacle and connected with it via two chutes. The base of the squatting slab can be either a stone-filled vault as shown above or a mound as indicated on figures 22 and 24. The chute and the flap trap are described on page 72.

The squatting slab can be cast directly on top of the stone-filled base or mound whichever is the case. The covers are best made of ferrocement, see page 91.

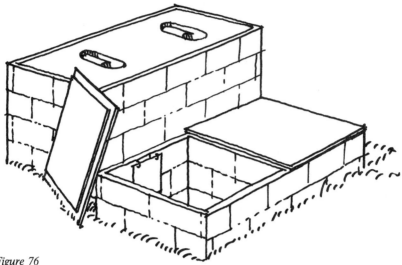

Figure 76

To make full use of the solar heat the latrine should be
oriented so that the covers receive as much sun as possible
and they should preferably be painted black.

FINAL DEPOSIT SYSTEMS
The ventilated pit latrine

Where soil and groundwater conditions permit a final deposit
system you should choose an improved type of pit latrine
rather than the traditional one illustrated on page 51. Either
a ventilated latrine as described below or a R.O.E.C. type as
described on page 101 - 105.

Start by marking the exact location of the pit, in this case
1 m square. Most soils require some stabilization of the
edges of the pit to prevent collapse. Before digging the pit
you should therefore make a concrete frame.

Dig a shallow trench, 60-80 mm deep, outside the 1 x 1 m

square marking the location of the pit. The trench serves as a form for the frame. Its width depends on the stability of the soil but should be at least 0.3 m, preferably more.

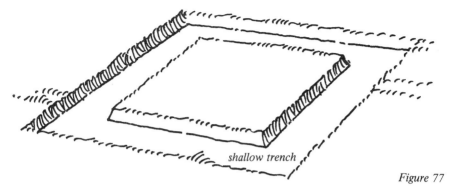

shallow trench

Figure 77

Mix some concrete and cover the bottom of the shallow trench with a layer 20-30 mm thick. On top of this place right away two reinforcement bars as shown in the figure below. The reinforcement bars should have a diameter of 8 mm or more. Place another layer of concrete, the same thickness as before, on top of the reinforcement.

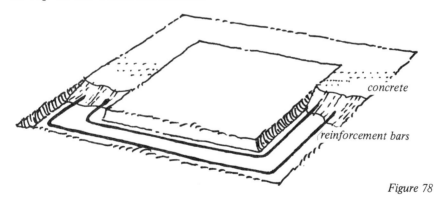

concrete

reinforcement bars

Figure 78

If reinforcement bars are not available, the frame can be made from timber as in figure 32.

After a day or two, start digging the pit inside the concrete frame. Make the pit as deep as possible - the deeper it is, the longer it will last. But keep clear of the ground water.

Not even in the rainy season must the ground water flood the pit.

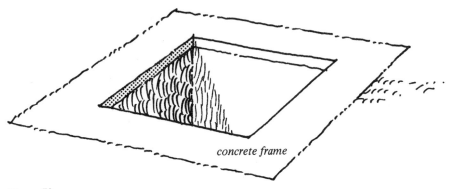

Figure 79

The squatting slab can be placed directly on the concrete frame but it is better to raise it above ground as shown below. Any kind of weather resistant building blocks can be used. In some locations it is even possible to use timber as shown in figure 34.

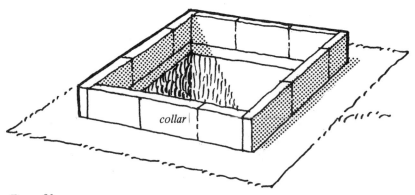

Figure 80

Make a squatting slab 1.1 x 1.1 m from ferrocement as described on page 91. As this slab is larger than the one used for a compost latrine it should be made thicker, say 22 mm. Use four layers of chicken-wire mesh as reinforcement.

98

Place the slab in position|

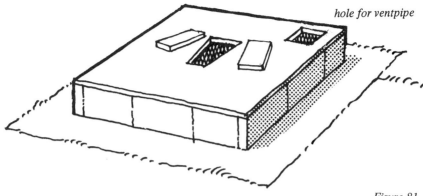

hole for ventpipe

Figure 81

and continue the masonry work until the superstructure, including the flue, is completed.

Add a stepping stone, door, roof, and, on top of the flue, a mosquito screen.

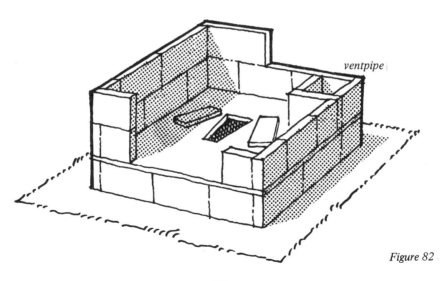

ventpipe

Figure 82

99

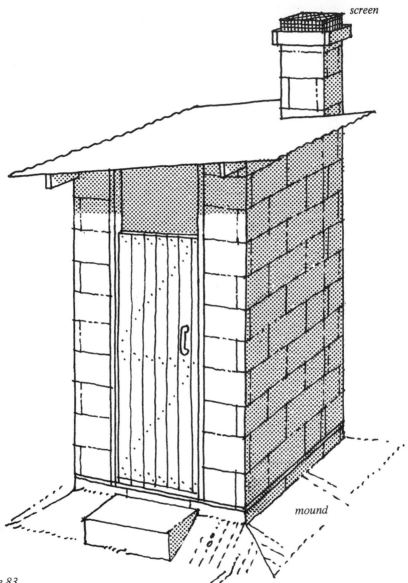

screen

mound

Figure 83

Put several layers of well tampered earth around the latrine
so that rain water is drained away.

100

The modified R.O.E.C.

The second of the pit latrines described here takes up quite
a lot of space on the ground: you need an area of about 2 x 3 m.
Start by marking out the exact location of the receptacle,
1.0 x 2.0 m.

Before digging the pit you should make a frame around it as
described on page 97   and in the following figures.

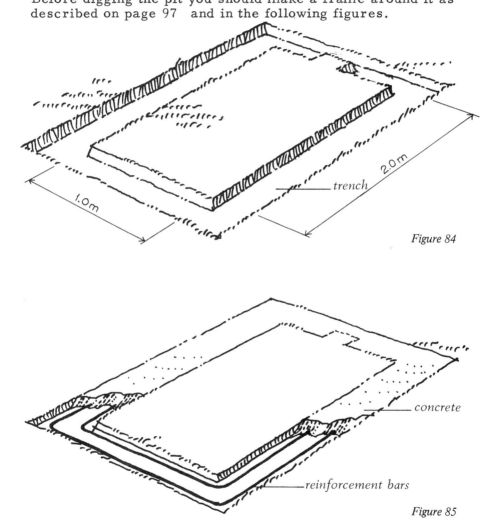

1.0 m

2.0 m

trench

Figure 84

concrete

reinforcement bars

Figure 85

When the frame is ready and the concrete has set, after a day or two, start digging the pit inside the concrete frame.

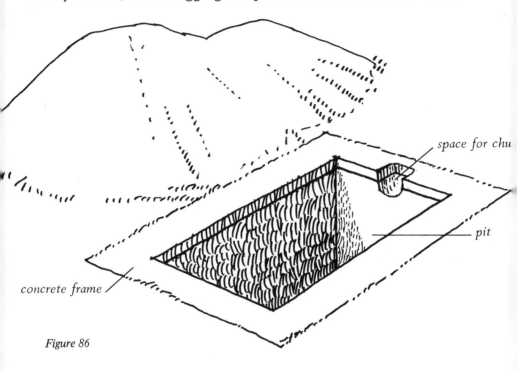

space for chu

pit

concrete frame

Figure 86

Any kind of building blocks could be used for the masonry construction. The concrete blocks in the figures opposite are the 50 x 190 x 390 mm ones mentioned earlier. For lining the pit it is necessary to use blocks with a thickness of 100 mm or more.

The squatting slab should be cast *in situ* and shaped into a bowl around the upper part of the chute. The lower part of the the chute should be provided with a flap-trap, see figure 103 opposite and also figure 52.

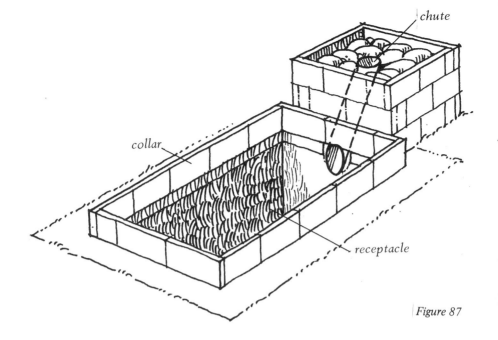

chute

collar

receptacle

Figure 87

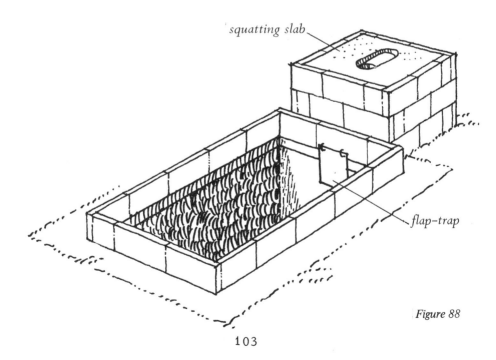

squatting slab

flap–trap

Figure 88

103

The cover over the receptacle could be made from ferrocement as described on page 91. Make it in three sections.
The one closest to the squatting slab should be provided with
a hole for the flue and a lid-covered manhole for inspection
of the flap-trap.

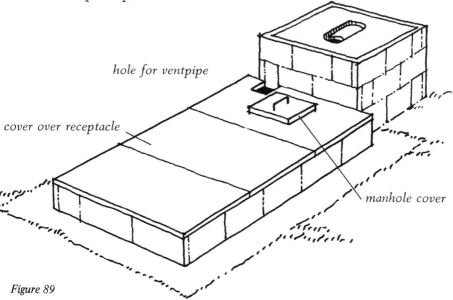

hole for ventpipe

cover over receptacle

manhole cover

Figure 89

Covers and lids must be completely fly-tight. This can be
achieved in several ways: the covers and the lids can be
made with a rim, all joints can be sealed with lime mortar
or the receptacle could be covered with a thick layer of
earth. The last method is illustrated on the figure opposite
which shows the latrine complete with flue and superstructure.

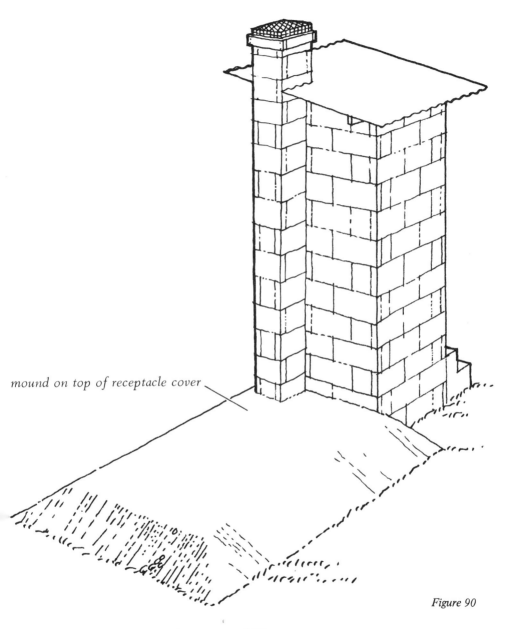

mound on top of receptacle cover

Figure 90

105

LATRINE AND BATH

Every house with a latrine should also have a separate enclosure for ablution purposes. It should be built at the same time as the latrine and preferably near it. Without such an enclosure there is a risk that the latrine is used not only for evacuation and anal cleansing but also for taking showers. A compost latrine rapidly turns into a stinking cesspool if large amounts of water are poured into the receptacle. A pit latrine is also likely to function better if its contents are not soaking wet.

The figure opposite shows a double-vault latrine with a bath enclosure attached. In the case of a pit latrine, drainage of bath water must be away from the pit.

Proper drainage is as essential as keeping the receptacle dry. Any accumulation of waste water can turn into a breeding ground for *Culex* mosquitoes.

An excellent material for the soakpit is charcoal. If this is not available, the soakpit should be filled with stones. In both cases a layer of gravel should be spread on top.

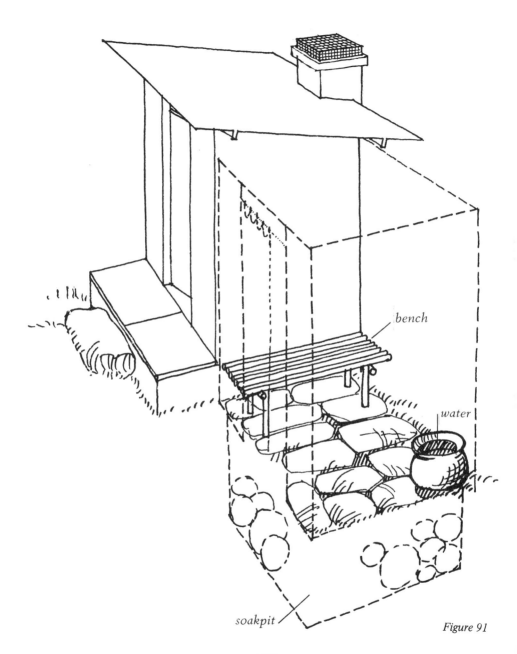

bench

water

soakpit

Figure 91

107

A multi-unit compost latrine

The preliminary version of this book dealt exclusively with latrines for single households. Many readers have, however, asked for advice on how to build communal latrines at schools, clinics and similar institutions located in areas where water is too precious to be flushed away through a WC.

The problem with public or communal facilities is not so much how to design and build a latrine, but rather how to keep it clean and how to operate it properly. The R.O.E.C. type, for instance, can without any design alterations be used as a public latrine.

Compost latrines, like any other type, must be cleaned frequently and in addition they require a daily input of organic refuse. Once or twice a year they must be emptied and users have to shift from one chamber to the other. Somebody must be in charge of these operations. If this can be arranged, compost latrines can be used as communal units.

The following figures illustrate one suitable combination of components. Four double-vault units have been combined and would probably cater for 40-50 people. (The solar heat collector increases the capacity of the latrine as compared to an ordinary latrine without heating device.)

The flue is essential for fly and odour control. One fluepipe serves two chambers, which means that the latrine illustrated here has four fluepipes.

A urinal should be built near the men's latrine. The urine could be collected, dilluted and used as a fertilizer or, if this is not feasible, drained away in a soakpit. Less urine in the receptacle means less need for organic refuse which in turn would give us a longer retention time.

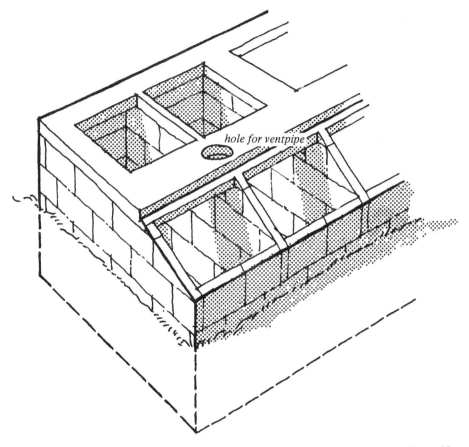

hole for ventpipe

Figure 92

Part of a multi-unit latrine.

109

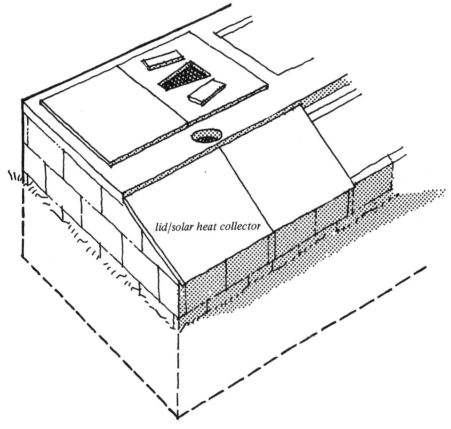

lid/solar heat collector

Figure 93

Same unit as in figure 92, now fitted with squatting slab, receptacle cover and solar heat collectors.

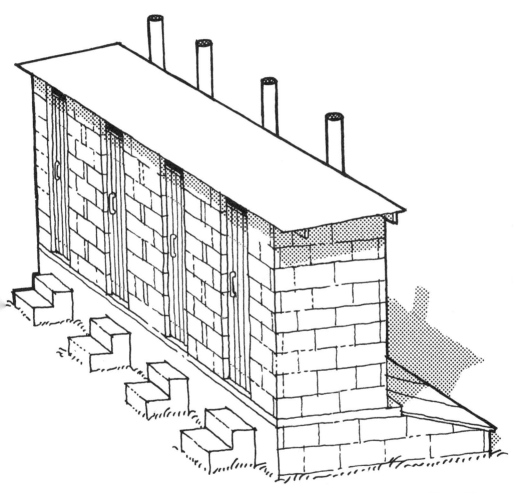

The multi-unit compost latrine completed.   *Figure 94*

111

Chapter 6

OPERATING INSTRUCTIONS

The construction of a latrine is only the first step. Proper use, careful upkeep and adequate disposal of the contents are equally important.

The adult user should have some knowledge of the relation between locally prevalent infectious diseases and excreta and she or he must have a basic understanding of the decomposition process. Every latrine construction programme must therefore be accompanied by a vigorous health education campaign.

The operating instructions in this chapter are primarily intended for those who use compost latrines but should be followed also by those who have pit latrines. Any traditional pit latrine or R.O.E.C. unit will function better if it is managed like a compost latrine. It is more likely to remain dry, the decomposition will be quicker and more complete, and odours and fly breeding will be reduced.

STARTING UP

Before the latrine is used for the first time the receptacle should be filled with losely packed organic residue: grass, weeds, leaves, straw, husks, sawdust, yard sweepings - whatever is available. This serves to absorb liquid, provides carbon for the decomposition, increases the variety of micro-organisms and prevents the pile from becoming too compact.

UTENSILS AND MATERIALS

Inside the latrine shelter there should be a brush for sweeping the squatting slab. Do not use this brush for any other purpose. Place a box or a jar full of ashes, husks, sawdust, dry earth or a mixture of such materials in a corner of the latrine shelter.

An empty tin or a coconut shell should be kept in the box to facilitate sprinkling of the dry material. If water is used for cleaning the anus, a bucket of water should always be kept in the shelter together with a tin for scooping it up.

DAILY USE

The number of regular users must be related to the capacity of the latrine. The capacity depends not only on the volume of the receptacle but to a great extent also on the input and on the climate.

A "gopuri" type of latrine with a vault size of 700 litres, and with input consisting of faeces, urine, water from anal cleansing, kitchen residues and sweepings, may work well for six to eight people. A Vietnam latrine with a vault size less than half that of the "gopuri", and input of faeces and ashes only, may serve up to ten persons.

Do not overload a compost latrine! The result will be a soggy mess, extremely unpleasant to clean out. If the receptacle is the final depository (traditional pit latrine, ventilated pit latrine or R.O.E.C.) overuse will drastically reduce the life of the latrine.

Use the latrine for excreting purposes only, not as a bathroom!

Sprinkle ashes, husks or powdered earth after each defecation.

Replace the lid.

When the slab becomes soiled: sprinkle with ashes and sweep into the receptacle. If water is used, use sparingly!

114

REGULAR UPKEEP

Put into the receptacle, preferably every day, all floor and yard sweepings as well as kitchen left overs.

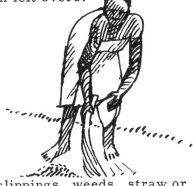

Figure 95

Several times a week put grass clippings, weeds, straw or leaves in the receptacle. Do not worry about filling it up too fast. The volume of whatever organic material you put in will in the end be reduced by 95%.

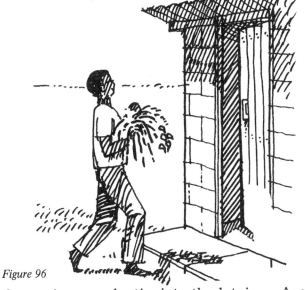

Figure 96

Do not throw glass, tins or plastic into the latrine. Avoid also slowly degradable materials such as corncobs, sugar canes, mango kernels and wooden sticks.

Save up the ashes and put them in the box mentioned previously, for later use in the latrine. The ashes deodorize the excreta, make the faecal matter less attractive to flies and absorb moisture.

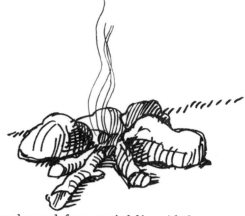

Figure 97

All husks should be saved and used for sprinkling if there are not enough ashes for this purpose. If not required for sprinkling, they can be dumped directly into the receptacle.

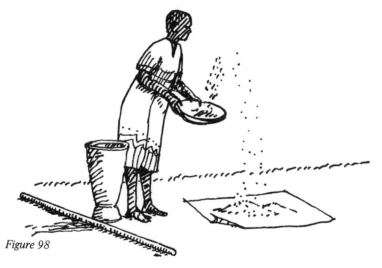

Figure 98

If there is a bucket of water for anal cleansing, make sure that the bucket is cleaned and emptied regularly, at least once every week, to prevent mosquitoes from breeding in it.

116

CHANGING VAULTS

When the receptacle is filled to within 0.3 - 0.4 m from the slab it is time to switch over to the other vault (or dig a new pit in the case of a pit latrine).

The pile should be covered with grass and topped up with soil. The vault should be closed with a heavy lid - either a special lid made from concrete or a piece of wood with a stone on top. The purpose of the heavy lid is to prevent any further use of this vault until the compost has been removed. Prepare the second receptacle as described under "Starting up" earlier in this chapter.

REMOVING COMPOST

When the second receptacle is nearly full it is time to remove the compost from the first one. Take off the cover and scoop up the contents with a hoe. All of it should not be removed - leave some to give the new pile a good start.

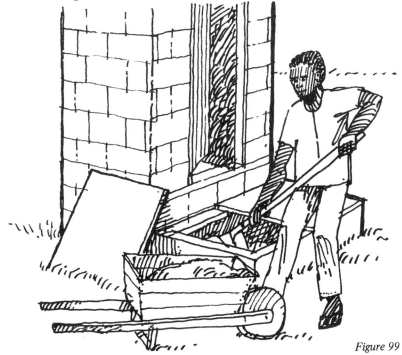

Figure 99

117

The compost should by now be fairly dry, soil like and completely odourfree. It is certainly not sterile but should be no more dangerous to handle than the soil in the garden.

Carry the compost to the vegetable plot or nearest field and put it in a shallow trench.

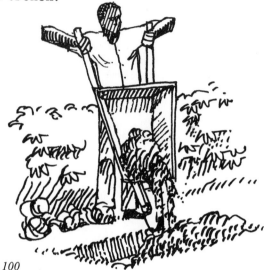

Figure 100

Cover it with about 0.1 m of soil.

MAINTENANCE

A "maintenance free" excreta disposal system does not exist. The simple, self-built latrines advocated in this book may require a great deal of maintenance. But they all have the advantage that they can be repaired by the users themselves. They are simple enough to require only the skills and materials readily available in the community.

Two things are specially important: Keep out surface water and make sure the receptacle is fly-tight.

The ground around the latrine must be arranged so that surface water drains away from the receptacle. Soil erosion may

118

change the direction of the flow. Check this during the rainy season.

Openings must be screened, holes and cracks repaired, and lids and covers must be tight fitting. A fly needs but a tiny crack to escape from the receptacle.

FLY CONTROL

Introduction of latrines in an area is likely to lead to an increased fly population because latrines provide an excellent breeding ground for various types of filth flies. These flies also breed in garbage, manure and dead animals. Odours from the latrine attract flies from a distance. If they manage to get inside the receptacle, the high moisture content of the faecal material there stimulates the fly to lay her eggs.

The adult fly can transmit infectious organisms in a number of ways: by the sticky hairs of its feet, by the hairs of its body, by regurgitation of its vomit drops and by its faeces. Diseases that can be transmitted by these flies include typhoid fever, the paratyphoids, cholera, bacillary dysentery, infantile diarrhoea, trachoma, poliomyelitis, yaws, amoebic dysentery and giardiasis. Certain worms can also be transmitted by flies (West 1951).

Latrines must therefore be constructed and operated in such a way that disease transmission is prevented. This can be done either by denying the flies access to faeces or by preventing them from leaving the receptacle.

We shall here describe and comment on a number of methods of fly control and point out which ones can be used for the types of latrines we are recommending. The various control measures have been grouped under the headings "mechanical", "thermal", "chemical", and "biological".

MECHANICAL CONTROL

Keeping the receptacle dark is often advocated as a fly control measure. It is advisable to do so - since flies are attracted by light - but it is certainly not enough. Flies do breed in dark pit latrines, in borehole types as well as in R.O.E.C. units, although both are supposedly "fly proof".

Professor Jettmar (1940) claimed that "it is mere superstition that latrine flies do not bree in deep and dark borehole latrines".

A latrine hole must have a lid. It is a minimum requirement but on its own it is far from enough. Flies do get in while the latrine is being used and some of the kitchen residues deposited in a compost latrine may already be flyblown. A self-closing device like the flap-trap described in Chapter 4 is more efficient than a hand operated lid.

Screening the latrine building is sometimes recommended but the effect is doubtful as in practice it is almost impossible to have it done and maintained properly. Besides, it does not work well for compost latrines for reasons mentioned above.

A screened ventpipe acts as a fly-trap if properly designed, see page 52 and the figure below. This kind of trap is self-cleaning and will automatically deposit the dead flies into the pit.

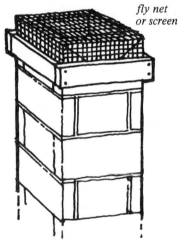

fly net or screen

Figure 101

If you want to use the dead flies as chicken feed you can make a trap from an empty kerosene tin and a piece of mosquito net as in the figure opposite. The trap has to be emptied frequently - maybe twice a week in the fly season. (While the trap is being emptied the hole must be covered!)

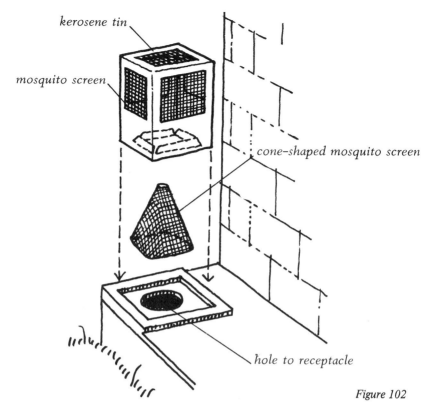

kerosene tin

mosquito screen

cone-shaped mosquito screen

hole to receptacle

Figure 102

In the vicinity of the latrine you can use freestanding fly-traps
made from kerosene tins as above or from timber and
mosquito net as in the figures on next page. A freestanding
trap has to be baited. Use animal intestines, manure or,
best of all, yeast. (Mix with water, allow mixture to stand
3-4 days with loosely sealed lid. Renew the bait after 3-5
days.) (Satrom 1979)

Fly swatters are useful tools in fly control inside houses,
especially in combination with screening.

However, the most efficient measure under this heading of
"mechanical control" is for each latrine user to sprinkle
liberal amounts of ashes, lime, sawdust, husks, peat or
dry earth over the faecal matter. Flies do not lay eggs in
any material with a moisture content of less than 65%.

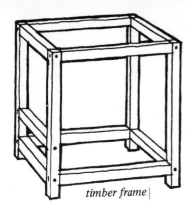

timber frame

A freestanding fly-trap, see also page 123.

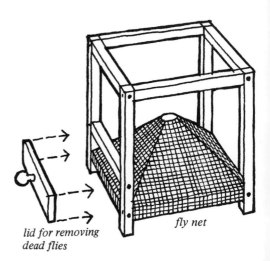

lid for removing dead flies

fly net

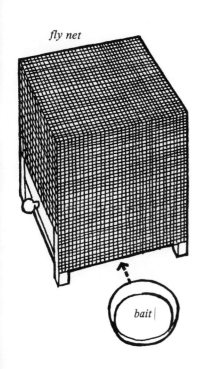

fly net

bait

Figure 103

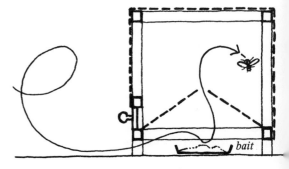

bait

THERMAL CONTROL

Thermal death of flies is not usually accomplished in a compost latrine - temperatures are too low. When lethal temperatures (above 49°C for adult flies) are reached inside a pile, the surface temperatures may still be tolerable to maggots. They are in any case able to move to cooler parts of the receptacle. The eggs are more succeptible - they cannot move and are more sensitive to high temperatures than larvae and pupae. Eggs will hatch at 40°C, some will survive at 41°C, but none at 43°. The exact lethal temperature depends also on the duration of the exposure (West 1951).

Pile surface temperatures can be increased by solar heating of the receptacle as described in Chapter 4. In most of the tropics it should be possible, with quite simple arrangements, to increase pile surface temperatures to 43°C or above.

Daily burning is a useful control measure for military latrines. Hay or straw is thrown into the pit and a sprinkling of crude oil added and the whole pile set on fire. Outside a military establishment the method might be used for temporary latrines in, for instance, refugee camps. For permanent latrines and household size units the method cannot be recommended as it is difficult to ensure that the burning is carried out regularly. Besides, not only flies but also many useful organisms would be destroyed by the fire.

Fly maggot destruction with chemicals was tried by Professor Jettmar in China in 1938. He came to the conclusion that the best method of killing larvae on a large scale was to use not chemicals but hot water. A large amount of boiling water suddenly poured over the surface of the latrine mass instantly kills all fly larvae (Jettmar 1940). The method is applied in boreholes but should certainly not be used in compost latrines!

CHEMICAL CONTROL

Fly breeding can be prevented by keeping the receptacle filled with smoke. The method is best suited for large, specially designed latrines like the one illustrated below (van Riel 1965).

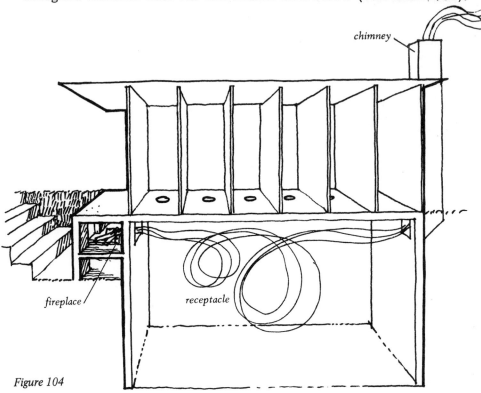

chimney

fireplace

receptacle

Figure 104

A variation of this method, at one time used for military latrines in East Africa, was to keep a smoking woodfire in a perforated kerosene tin suspended halfway down the pit by wires. It was necessary to renew the fire twice a day.

In the early days of DDT usage, effective control was achieved in several parts of the world. Nowadays lasting results cannot be expected from the use of chemical insecticides. The housefly has a short life cycle and quickly develops resistance against chemicals. The enemies of the fly are also affected by the insecticide but are not able to develop resistance as fast as the fly. The end result of using insecticides against the housefly is therefore an increase in the fly population as well as a destruction of desirable organisms. Insecticides are toxic to man - when used persistently there is a risk that

ground water and soil will be polluted. An additional disadvantage of chemical insecticides is that they are too expensive for most fly infested communities in developing countries.
In short: insecticides cannot be relied upon for fly control in
latrines.

Experimental work on the use of synthetic hormones in preventing the growth of flies in manure has been carried out in
the US (Anon., 1975). The hormones, similar to some insect
hormones, are incorporated in the feed of cattle and chickens
and permeate the manure. When tested on four of the most
important species of flies they proved 100% effective, The
hormones have been derived from terpene chemicals with a
relatively simple manufacturing process. There are no
reports on what might happen to humans who consume the
products of the cattle and chickens fed on hormones. If the
hormones were also to permeate the human faeces this would
open up a completely new prospect for fly control in latrines.

BIOLOGICAL CONTROL

In all latrines there is naturally a certain amount of biological
control of the fly population. The most obvious one is carried
out by reptiles. Lizards and chameleons are great devourers
of flies and a latrine and its immediate surroundings is one of
their favourite locations. Lizards often live inside the receptacle. Spiders may be even more important and in many
latrines the space between the pile and the squatting slab is
filled with spider webs. Frogs can also easily survive in a
compost latrine.

Less obvious but equally or more important is the biological
control carried out by tiny fly parasites, pathogens and pre-
dators. Several species can be released in the fly breeding
area where they live on fly eggs and larvae. The most widely
used are *Tachenandphagus zelandicus*, *Spalangia indus* and
Mucidifurax raptor (Parker 1977).

T. zelandicus is native to New Zealand and Australia. It can
lay 5-10 eggs in a single maggot. The immature stages of the
life cycle lasts 22 days at 21°C and the adult lives 8 to 15 days.

S. indus is a hot weather parasite native to California. It attacks the fly pupae, puncturing the outer pupal wall. Its immature life cycle is 22 days at 27°C and the adult lives 30 to 40 days. *M. raptor* is similar to *S. indus* in activity.

Agriculturalists have for many years known that several of the rod-shaped bacilli are insect pathogens. The bacilli concerned cause fatal disease in the larvae of certain insects, including the housefly and the mosquito.

Bacillus thuringiensis has proved effective against fly breeding in stables, pigstries, chicken coops and manure piles. These bacilli might also be effective for fly control in compost and pit latrines (Carlberg 1979).

CONCLUSIONS

No one measure alone is likely to achieve complete fly control. For pit and compost latrines in developing countries action should be based on a combination of the following methods:

> a lid, preferably a self-closing flap-trap; all other openings to the receptacle must be screened and holes and cracks immediately repaired;

> the user should sprinkle ashes, lime, husks or powdered earth over each deposit of faeces;

> lizards, frogs, spiders and *B. thuringiensis* should be encouraged to live and multiply in the receptacle.

In addition, whenever possible, compost latrines should be constructed with a simple solar heat collector over the receptacle.

REFERENCES CITED

ANONYMOUS (1975), Killing flies with hormones, Ceres **8** (4):67

CARLBERG, G. (1976), Biologisk bekämpning av skadeinsekter, Finlands natur **35** (3):3–6

JETTMAR, H. M. (1940), Some experiments on the resistance of the latrine fly, *Chrysomyia megacephala,* against chemicals, Chinese Medical Journal **57**:74-85.

PARKER, J. L. (1977), Agressive little parasites will dine on fly larvae, Countryside, **61**(6):40.

van RIEL, J. (1965), *Santé publique tropicale,* Éditions Desoer, Liège, Belgium.

SATROM, G. & STEPHENS, D. (1979), *A fly control handbook,* (mimeo), Beneficial Biosystems Inc, 1603 63rd St, Emeryville, Ca 94608, USA.

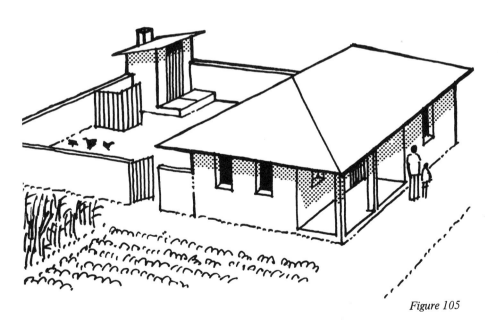

Figure 105

129

INDEX